The
Mitral Valve Prolapse Syndrome/Dysautonomia Survival Guide

James F. Durante

Cheryl L. Durante

John G. Furiasse, MD

Foreword by Phillip C. Watkins, MD, FACC

New Harbinger Publications, Inc.

Publisher's Note

Distributed in the U.S.A. by Publishers Group West; in Canada by Raincoast Books; in Great Britain Hi Marketing Ltd.; in South Africa by Real Books, Ltd.; in Australia by Boobook; and in New Zealand by Tandem Press.

Copyright © 2002 by James F. Durante, Cheryl L. Durante, and John G. Furiasse
New Harbinger Publications, Inc.
5674 Shattuck Avenue
Oakland, CA 94609

Cover design by Lightbourne Images
Edited by Kayla Sussell
Text design by Michele Waters

ISBN 1-57224-303-1 Paperback

New Harbinger Publications' Web site address: www.newharbinger.com

04   03   02

10   9   8   7   6   5   4   3   2   1

First printing

Dedicated to our dad, Jim, the most unique father in the world, for being there for us twenty-four hours a day, seven days a week. Also, to the two Bonnies in our lives, who epitomize elegance and strength. We love you all dearly.

Contents

Foreword

For all too long, a large group of patients have had many symptoms that have been quite confusing both to them and to the medical profession. Over the years, these patients have been diagnosed with everything from hypoglycemia to chronic fatigue syndrome, fibromyalgia, anxiety, "thyroid problems," and so on. It is only in the past few years that we have become aware of what is actually happening with these patients. Not since Lyn Frederickson's book (1992) was written many years ago has information become available that will be of as much benefit to this large group of patients as the *Mitral Valve Prolapse Syndrome/Dysautonomia Survival Guide* will be.

In the past four or five years we have learned that this syndrome is actually a disorder of the autonomic nervous system. This is referred to as *Dysautonomia*. We now also understand why these patients have such diverse symptoms. They may complain of fatigue, which actually is the most common symptom that troubles them, but they also have very troubling cardiovascular symptoms.

These symptoms can range from chest pain severe enough to warrant a trip to the emergency room at times, to occasional, fleeting sharp pains. Along with this, palpitations or an irregular skipping heartbeat are very common. These may occur when the person is totally at rest with no exertion and, especially, at night when lying down.

Many of these patients, particularly the younger ones in their teenage years, experience spells of profound dizziness, weakness, the feeling of almost blacking out, and, at times, they do have episodes of passing out or fainting. We now understand how this is influenced by a low blood volume, a low blood pressure, and surges of adrenaline. Other symptoms of abnormal autonomic function may be present, such as irritable bowel syndrome (spastic colon), various vascular and migraine headache syndromes, cold extremities, and mood disorders. The mood disorders are particularly troubling, as these cause these patients to be identified as having psychological problems when, in fact, they have a physiological abnormality of the autonomic nervous system that, if left untreated, may indeed lead to psychological problems.

This book is truly a "Survivor's Guide" both for understanding why these unusual symptoms occur together, and for aid with seeking appropriate medical help and the proper lifestyle changes. Clearly, understanding and education go a long way to helping cope with this problem. It is certainly not a simple cardiovascular problem as it has so long been labeled with the term "mitral valve prolapse." It is more of a neurological/endocrine/dysautonomia abnormality.

This *Survivor's Guide* will become the baseline resource manual for those who wish to understand the disorder and want to know how to properly treat and manage it. This is a book that every physician should read. In it you will find in-depth explanations for these sets of symptoms, and very appropriate clinical information that will help to illustrate what is happening in the body when the symptoms are active.

This is a book that we will highly recommend to our patients as an instruction manual for dealing with this disorder of autonomic function that we now term Mitral Valve Prolapse Syndrome/Dysautonomia.

—Phillip C. Watkins, M.D., F.A.C.C.
Medical Director,
The Mitral Valve Prolapse/Dysautonomia Center
Birmingham, Alabama

Acknowledgments

This book would never have been written without the support of several very special people. Thank you Lyn and Dr. H for giving us back our quality of life. Lyn Frederickson was a pioneer in writing about mitral valve prolapse syndrome/dysautonomia. Had it not been for her book, this book would not have become a reality.

Dr. Mason, thank you for being so open-minded and willing to listen.

To Wayne, whose unwavering belief in us brought us to the point where we are today.

Finally, to Kayla, who taught us how to write a book and who went above and beyond her job of editing. It was a pleasure working with you.

Introduction

Mitral valve prolapse (MVP) is one of the most overdiagnosed, misdiagnosed, and misunderstood disorders in medicine. It runs the spectrum of asymptomatic stethoscope findings of MVP to full-blown Marfan's syndrome (an hereditary condition of connective tissue, bones, muscles, and ligaments that can result in a variety of medical problems).

So, you can see that the range of what is diagnosed as MVP is very broad indeed. At one end of the spectrum, a diagnosis of MVP may have no physical consequences other than a prolapsed mitral valve. In all other regards, the patient is asymptomatic and has no symptoms other than the click heard in the physician's stethoscope, which sound is produced by a prolapsed mitral valve.

At the other end of the spectrum, Marfan's syndrome sometimes results in a dilated aorta that becomes so weakened that an aneurysm develops. In between, there are a variety of symptoms ranging from dysautonomia to congestive heart failure.

The symptoms of mitral valve prolapse syndrome (MVPS) and dysautonomia are very similar, in some cases identical, and because the medical establishment has yet to settle on which term to use as standard nomenclature, the term MVPS/D is used throughout this text. The intention of this book is to shed light on MVP, MVPS, and dysautonomia. Through clinical vignettes the reader is introduced to individuals who have been afflicted with the many symptoms attributed to MVPS/D. In these stories, the reader will encounter first-hand accounts of how different individuals have suffered and dealt with this disorder.

Those afflicted with MVPS/D have often been frustrated with traditional medical care. They have frequently felt isolated and abandoned. Physicians, too, have been frustrated because of the lack of adequate diagnostic testing tools and effective treatments.

When confronted with repetitive complaints by patients, doctors often respond with simple avoidance, patronizing comments, such as "It's all in your head," or psychiatric referral. This occurs because of the lack of adequate diagnostic tests or medical treatments, and these physicians' avoidance of nontraditional treatments.

Patients who have encountered these kinds of responses from their doctors often fall in an abyss of hopelessness, fear, and depression. It is our hope that after finishing this book such a reader will have a better understanding of the testing and treatment modalities that are currently available to diagnose and treat those with MVPS/D.

My interest in this disorder and this book is more than just a professional one. My wife has dealt with a variety of the symptoms discussed in these chapters for the past twenty years. Many of the pains, frustrations, and fears described within have resonance in our lives. It is our hope that in addition to basic knowledge, this book will bring encouragement and hope to those afflicted with MVPS/D.

Finally, it is essential to understand that this book is not a substitute for a complete medical evaluation by a competent physician. Many people will self-diagnose themselves erroneously as having MVPS/D, only to be diagnosed with an entirely different condition when they are seen by competent physicians. It could be disastrous to avoid proper medical evaluation and treatment due to the false belief that you are suffering from MVPS/D.

With that caveat aside, when you turn the page, you will begin your journey into this family of disorders by first exploring the mitral valve, which is where this disease entity originates.

> —John G. Furiasse, M.D., F.A.C.C.,
> Director of Cardiac Rehabilitation
> Alexian Brothers Medical Center
> Elk Grove Village, Illinois

CHAPTER 1

Mitral Valve Prolapse and Mitral Valve Prolapse Syndrome

Illness opens doors to a reality that is closed to a healthy point of view.

—Anonymous

If you have picked this book up while browsing, there is a good likelihood that you have, think you have, or know someone who has mitral valve prolapse (MVP) or mitral valve prolapse syndrome (MVPS). If you were recently diagnosed with MVP, you may be quite confused, even frightened. You were probably told it is a benign condition, yet it may be difficult for you to understand how you can have something wrong with your heart and not have some type of cardiac disease. Equally confusing may be the fact that you sometimes experience palpitations and chest pain that you perceive as cardiac-related.

If you do decide to read this book, you will be taking a giant step in the right direction because information is always good, and the more information you have, the better equipped you will be to help yourself deal with any issues that either MVP or MVPS may bring into your life. So, now, what exactly is MVP? And how does MVPS differ from MVP? Let's deal with these two questions one step at a time.

The Heart of the Matter

First, take a look at figure 1. There you will see that the mitral valve is located in the heart between the left ventricle and the left atrium. It got its name because it resembles the shape of a bishop's hat or miter. The valve is quite small, measuring approximately 4.5 square centimeters or approximately one and three-quarter inches, about the size of a 50-cent coin. The purpose of the heart is to pump blood throughout the body. To accomplish that task, the heart is divided into four chambers, the left and right atria, and the left and right ventricles. There are two parts on each side of the heart separated by a wall-like divider called a septum. Normally, the right side of the heart has no communication with the left side.

The left side of the heart receives oxygenated blood from the lungs and pumps it to the tissues via the arteries. The right side of the heart receives deoxygenated blood via the veins, from the tissues, and pumps it to the lungs. Each side of the heart has two

Normal Mitral Valve

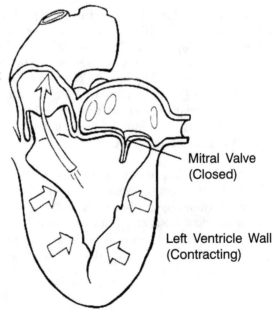

Normal Movement of Blood Through the Left Side of the Heart

Mitral Valve (Closed)

Left Ventricle Wall (Contracting)

Figure 1: Heart with a Closed Mitral Valve

valves. They are there to make sure blood flows through the heart with every beat. These valves are formed from strong flaps of tissue, called *leaflets* or *cusps*, that open and close as the heart pumps. They control how the blood travels.

For the system to work properly, the valves must open at the proper time, allow the blood to flow through the heart, and then close tightly, so that none of the blood flows backwards. It may help you to think of a properly functioning mitral valve as a one-way door. If the valve does not remain closed, that is, if it operates as a two-way door, the valve may "billow" back into the upper chamber (the left atrium). This can cause blood to leak back into the upper chamber.

Mitral Valve Prolapse

The mitral valve is one of the four valves in the heart. It is located on the left side between the left atrium and the left ventricle (see figure 1). The other three valves are called the *aortic, tricuspid,* and *pulmonary*. In a normal heart, when the lower part of the heart contracts, the mitral valve remains firm. When a mitral valve is somewhat looser than normal, one of its parts may "billow," or "flop" backward slightly into the upper chamber (the left atrium) during the heart's contraction. This is called a *prolapse* (see figure 2). A mitral valve prolapse is caused by a slight variation in the composition of the valve itself.

When one of the parts of the mitral valve billows or flops back, the "flopping" action can create a clicking sound that may or may not be heard with a stethoscope. Occasionally, when the valve is flopping, there will be slight leakage of blood (called *regurgitation*) that flows backwards into the upper chamber of the heart. This can be heard as a heart murmur.

Mitral valve prolapse is one of the most common cardiac findings. It appears to be genetically transmitted, but not everyone in an affected family will have the disorder. It seems to affect women three times more often than men (MVP Center 1989).

Mitral valve prolapse is a well-recognized clinical disorder with a reported prevalence in the total population of 4 to 18 percent. This wide range is caused by differences in age, gender, and ethnic background of those tested for the disorder, and also by different diagnostic criteria (Freed, Levy, Levine, Larson, et al. 1999). As stated above, it is believed to have a much higher incidence in women than in men.

Prolapsed Mitral Valve

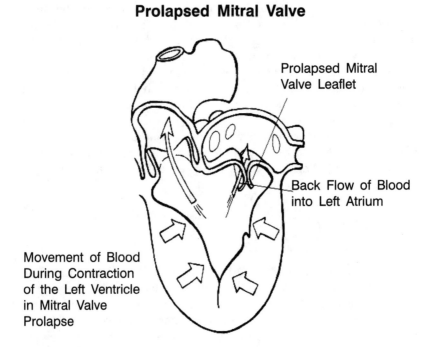

Prolapsed Mitral
Valve Leaflet

Back Flow of Blood
into Left Atrium

Movement of Blood
During Contraction
of the Left Ventricle
in Mitral Valve
Prolapse

Figure 2: Heart with a Prolapsed Mitral Valve

How MVP Is Discovered

Often, mitral valve prolapse is discovered during a routine stetho-scope examination of the heart. Unsettling as such a discovery may be at first, the condition is rarely a cause for concern. The tiny amount of extra motion, or the flexibility of the mitral valve in itself is not harmful and causes no damage to the heart or to the body. Few people with mitral valve prolapse exhibit any symptoms at all.

Prolapse means that the valve tends not to work with 100 per-cent efficiency, and some blood may flow backwards or "regurgi-tate" from the left ventricle to the left atrium. The exact amount of regurgitation varies from person to person. A cardiologist can deter-mine the specific amount. Although mitral regurgitation is the most significant complication of mitral valve prolapse, the majority of people have mild or no regurgitation (Mulumudi and Bivekananthan 2001).

In an extremely small percentage of cases, however, mitral valve prolapse can cause episodes of rapid heartbeat, chest pain, and significant valve leakage that may require regular medical attention or even surgery. The cumulative risk for valve replacement surgery for severe mitral regurgitation in people with mitral valve prolapse is estimated to be 2.6 percent in men and 0.8 percent in women before age sixty-five. By age seventy-five, the same risk in men and women becomes 5.5 percent and 1.4 percent, respectively (Singh, Cappuci, Kramer-Fox, Roman, Kligfield, et al. 2000). If you happen to be one of these very rare cases, your physician will know this from the results of your diagnostic tests.

Diagnosing Mitral Valve Prolapse

Diagnostic tests help to rule out serious heart disease by demonstrating how well your heart is pumping and how your valves are working. The test most often used to detect mitral valve prolapse is called the echocardiogram (ECHO), or cardiogram ultrasonography. The test is painless and involves no risk. Before you take it, you are asked to remove the clothing from your upper body. You may be asked to lie on your left side and possibly on your back. During the test, a technician moves a small device called a transducer (lubricated with gel) over various places on your chest. The transducer picks up the beating of your heart and sends the information to the computer. The sound waves coming from your heart create patterns that are then amplified as three-dimensional images on a computer screen. These images display the structure and movements of your heart's valves and chambers.

When you have an echocardiogram, you also may have an EKG, or electrocardiogram, simultaneously. The EKG is a test that records electrical signals from your heart onto a paper strip. To perform this test, electrodes are attached to your wrists, ankles, and chest, through adhesive strips that conduct electrical impulses.

The electrical signals form a pattern on the paper strip that may offer clues to your physician that there may be an underlying problem with your heart, such as heart damage, an arrhythmia, or an electrical problem. After obtaining the necessary information, the technician will remove the transducer and electrodes and send the test results to your physician.

Another common method for detecting mitral valve prolapse is to have a cardiologist listen for a "click" through a stethoscope. The click should be sought with the patient in three separate positions: lying down, seated, and standing.

False Positives and False Negatives

Keep in mind that if an ECHO test is interpreted as not showing definite mitral valve prolapse, that should not rule out its presence. There can be a wide variability in the techniques used by the technician and also in the physician's interpretation. Note, too, that mitral valve prolapse often is more easily observed when the patient sits in an upright position during the recording of the test.

Furthermore, some tests indicate that when someone is even slightly dehydrated when taking the test, there is a greater chance of a positive result, even if the person does not have MVP. This is called a "false positive." The contrary situation is also true. Someone who is very well hydrated may have a negative result on the test, and still have MVP. This is called a "false negative." It is essential for you and your doctor to look at all of the elements of the entire picture before making a diagnosis of MVP.

Mitral Valve Infection

People with a prolapsed mitral valve and a leaking, or regurgitating, valve are at slightly higher risk than the rest of the population of contracting a bacterial heart infection called *endocarditis*. This is an inflammation of the membranes of the heart. In this condition, there is a very slight risk during certain medical procedures that bacteria may be released into the bloodstream that can lodge in the prolapsing mitral valve and result in infection. For this reason, many physicians recommend taking antibiotics beforehand for certain dental and medical procedures. The various antibiotics used as safeguards for these procedures include amoxicillin, ampicillin, clindamycin, cephalexin, azithromycin, gentamicin, and vancomycin. Note that there are many other physicians who do not recommend taking antibiotics for those procedures. If someone has only structural MVP without a leaking, regurgitating valve, they believe the risk of infection is so low that it does not justify the risk of an allergic reaction to antibiotics.

Endocarditis is very rare, but it can be difficult to treat. Among all people with mitral valve prolapse, the occurrence of infective endocarditis is 32 cases per million dental procedures; among people with a heart murmur, the incidence is 78 cases per million dental procedures (Devereux, Frary, Kramer-Fox, Isom, Borer, Roman, et al. 1994). If you have been diagnosed with mitral valve prolapse, be sure to discuss this issue thoroughly with your physician regarding his or her recommendations.

Procedures That May Require Antibiotics

- All dental procedures likely to induce gum bleeding

- Tonsillectomy or adenoidectomy

- Surgical procedures or biopsies involving the respiratory system

- Bronchoscopy

- Incision and drainage of infected tissue, such as an abscess

- Procedures involving the urinary tract, such as a cystoscopy

- Procedures involving the esophagus, stomach, or bowel (endoscopy)

- Vaginal gynecological procedures

- Gallbladder surgery

Mitral Valve Prolapse Syndrome

There is a certain amount of confusion regarding the differences between mitral valve prolapse (MVP) and mitral valve prolapse syndrome (MVPS). So, let's see if we can clear up that difference for you right now. It is true that MVP is usually described as a structural, but not life-threatening, defect in the heart. As mentioned above, it is a defect thought to be genetically determined; so, usually, it is found in families.

The diagnosis of MVPS is not so straightforward and, in fact, there is a certain amount of controversy and confusion about the many different symptoms that are associated with the condition. Some people believe that the syndrome is comprised of two different conditions: mitral valve prolapse and MVP-associated dysautonomia. They believe that, when these two conditions occur together, they make up mitral valve prolapse syndrome.

Despite years of research, the symptomatology and significance of MVP and MVPS remains debatable. Researchers disagree as to whether these two distinct conditions even exist. Although the medical community is gradually coming around, many physicians still believe MVPS is a current "fad" in medicine that has no clinical significance. Too often patients are viewed as "too worried" while the physician "blows off" the patient's symptoms, leading to friction in the patient/doctor relationship. A physician once remarked, "Barring discovery of hard evidence for some causal link between them

(MVP and dysautonomia), I'm inclined to the view that the overlap between the conditions is coincidental" (Abben, no date).

Many people with mitral valve prolapse appear to have a more reactive or hypersensitive autonomic nervous system than normal. This has led some researchers to call this imbalance mitral valve prolapse syndrome (MVPS) or Dysautonomia (dysfunction of the autonomic nervous system). In any case, it doesn't really matter which name you use regarding MVPS; the symptoms are very real and very distressing.

What Is a Syndrome?

Webster defines a syndrome as a group of signs and symptoms that occur together and are characteristic of a specific disorder. Mitral valve prolapse syndrome (MVPS) is characterized by dizziness, numbness, chest pain, anxiety, sleeplessness, fatigue, mood swings, and numerous other symptoms. How can a mitral valve prolapse cause such a variety of symptoms?

The answer is that these symptoms are not caused by the prolapse of the mitral valve itself. The prolapse of the mitral valve is actually just a marker, or an identifier, for someone who exhibits this complex of symptoms. *The prolapse is not the prime cause of the symptoms.*

The symptoms are caused by an imbalance in a part of the central nervous system (CNS) called the autonomic nervous system (ANS). The ANS is the fine-tuning mechanism of the body and it is responsible for the balance of virtually every bodily function there is. Some of the most important functions the autonomic nervous system governs are these: heart rate, blood pressure, digestive functions, body temperature and perspiration, sleep patterns, bladder and bowel functions, constriction or dilation of the eyes' pupils, lung functions, reproductive organs, adrenaline output, and sexual reflexes.

Jill's Story

When Jill began suffering from panic attacks and chest pains at the age of twenty-eight, at first she thought she was dying. Several months later, she started experiencing sleeplessness, dizziness, and heart palpitations. Although she thought she was very ill and most likely dying, everyone in her family thought she was just a world-class hypochondriac.

That was more than four years ago. Now, five physicians and several thousand dollars later, she knows she is not dying, but she also knows that she does have a disorder that can make its sufferer believe otherwise—MVPS. Today, Jill has made her peace with the syndrome, and she has made the necessary changes to her lifestyle so as not to worry when she experiences any of the symptoms (see chapters 9 and 11).

Among those who have MVPS, women tend to have the more severe symptoms. The age of the onset of symptoms ranges broadly between the teens and the mid-forties, but a few people both younger and older have been noted in the literature (Davies 1995). The typical person with severe symptoms is a woman between twenty-five and forty-five years of age who has been having at least mild symptoms for several years. Frequently, she has consulted a number of physicians without receiving a diagnosis.

Here is what we know about mitral valve prolapse syndrome to date: a structural prolapse of the mitral valve does not cause it, but it is associated with mitral valve prolapse. If you have a prolapsed valve leaflet, that is an indicator that you may have, or are predisposed to have, mitral valve prolapse syndrome. There appears to be an excellent reason to call this complex of symptoms mitral valve prolapse syndrome/dysautonomia (MVPS/D) to indicate there is far more involved than the small amount of prolapse of the mitral valve leaflet.

Conditions That Mimic MVPS/D

There are several conditions that present many of the same symptoms as MVPS/D, hence, in this book, they are called MVPS/D mimickers. These conditions are as follows:

- Hypoglycemia

- Thyroid disorder

- Chronic fatigue syndrome

- Bipolar disorder (manic-depression)

- Exercise-induced asthma

- Hyperventilation

- ADD (attention deficit disorder)

Physical Commonalties in MVP and MVPS/D

Often, people with MVP or MVPS/D exhibit specific types of variations in their skeletal structure. That is to say that certain physical characteristics are common among those with MVP or MVPS/D. Here are some of those characteristics:

- Marfanoid habitus: This term is used to describe the tall, usually lanky, thin body shape. It is frequently accompanied by features like hyperextensible joints or thin, "spidery" fingers.

- Micromastia: This term is used to describe smaller than normal female breasts, especially when the patient is compared with other women in her family who do not have MVP or MVPS/D.

- Straight back syndrome: This term is used to describe curvature of the spine, where the upper body sways backward. It is also known as "swayback" or "lordosis." The thoracic spine (the middle part of the spine) is abnormally straight in the upper back.

- Scoliosis: This is curvature of the spine.

- Pectus excavatum: This is a congenital condition in which the sternum (breastbone) is abnormally depressed. It is also known as "sunken breastbone."

- Cervical rib syndrome: In this condition there is an extra rib located in the area of the neck. It sometimes develops in connection with a cervical (neck) vertebra, usually the lowest vertebra.

History of Mitral Valve Prolapse Syndrome/Dysautonomia

Don't be surprised if many people, including some physicians, are unfamiliar with the syndrome of MVPS/D. When we look back into history it becomes clear that it has been around for decades, but it had other names attached to it in the past: These include "irritable heart," "soldier's heart," "Barlow's Syndrome," and "DaCosta's Syndrome." It has also been speculated that many years ago, when people spoke of having the "vapors" or "swooning," they may have been speaking of the symptoms of MVPS/D.

Mitral valve prolapse syndrome/dysautonomia was first observed during the American Civil War among soldiers who experienced fatigue, shortness of breath, palpitations, and chest pain in response to the stress of combat. In fact, this so-called "irritable heart" became a reason to pull soldiers off the combat field. Somewhere between 1860 and 1870 Dr. Joseph DeCosta called the syndrome "irritable heart" and "disability in young soldiers" (Watkins 1990).

During the First World War, when British doctors observed severe exhaustion and extreme changes in soldiers' heart rates, they called the syndrome "soldier's heart" and "effort syndrome." In this same era, the syndrome was observed in civilians as well as in military personnel. After the war, during which time (1914-1917) more women had entered the workforce, many women began experiencing symptoms identical to those of the soldiers suffering from "effort syndrome." By 1941, a new label was invented to describe the problem: "anxiety neurosis." It is a matter of some interest that, just as soon as women began exhibiting the symptoms of "soldier's heart," the term "neurosis" came into use to describe the symptoms of the syndrome.

In the early 1960s, technological advances produced the echocardiogram, which allowed physicians to see the mitral valve in motion for the first time. This led them to the discovery that the clicking sound they had been hearing in stethoscope examinations was caused by the "flopping" mitral valve leaflet. From 1970 to 1980 it was referred to both as Barlow's syndrome and as its most enduring name, "mitral valve prolapse syndrome."

MVP and MVPS/D Are Two Separate Conditions

Many people refer to MVP and MVPS/D as if they were the same condition. Clearly, they are not. But for those who have been diagnosed only with mitral valve prolapse, this confusion in terms can lead to greater confusion in understanding. For example, if you have MVPS/D, people who have been diagnosed with MVP might tell you that they have the same condition you do, but they've never experienced any anxiety or panic attacks or anything remotely like that. In other words, they're saying to you, "Why do you have so many problems? You only have MVP. It's not such a big deal." They can say that because these people do not have MVPS/D.

But if you are on the receiving end of such comments, they may cause you to doubt yourself and to wonder if indeed there is something else wrong with you—something mental. Such confusion and the resultant worry and anxiety take place all the time, even among physicians.

Dysautonomia

For all of the reasons indicated above there is certainly good cause to call this complex of symptoms mitral valve prolapse syndrome/dysautonomia (MVPS/D), rather than simply mitral valve prolapse. The use of two different names for the two different conditions will certainly lessen the confusion. In recent years the term MVPS/D has been recognized as the most appropriate name for mitral valve prolapse syndrome (MVP Center 1990).

Hopefully, MVPS/D will be the exclusive term used in the future. In this book, it is the term that we use. We will discuss the features of dysautonomia in chapter 2. To sum up the major points discussed in this chapter (and for use as a handy reference) here is a list of the main differences between mitral valve prolapse and mitral valve prolapse syndrome/dysautonomia.

Mitral Valve Prolapse	Mitral Valve Prolapse Syndrome/Dysautonomia
• Prolapsed mitral valve	• Prolapsed mitral valve
• Possible regurgitation	• Possible regurgitation
• May be tall and lanky	• May be tall and lanky
• Spidery fingers	• Spidery fingers
• Hyperextensible joints (flexible)	• Hyperextensible joints (flexible)
• Scoliosis (curvature of the spine)	• Scoliosis (curvature of the spine)
• May suffer from palpitations	• Nervous system imbalance
	• Rapid heart rate
	• Palpitations
	• Chest pain

- Fatigue
- Headaches
- Irritable bowel syndrome (IBS)
- Gastroesophageal reflux (GERD)
- Dizziness
- Fibromyalgia
- Anxiety, panic attacks
- Mood swings
- Depression
- Sleep disorders
- PMS
- Shortness of breath
- Temporomandibular joint dysfunction (TMJ)
- Concentration or memory problems
- Twitching muscles, shakiness
- Numbness or tingling
- Visual disturbances
- Weakness
- Skin problems or rashes

CHAPTER 2

Dysautonomia

It is part of the cure, to wish to be cured.

—Hippolytus

It is believed that when the autonomic nervous system (ANS) is forming in the developing fetus (at approximately six weeks), the mitral valve is also being formed. Various researchers believe that 40 percent of those who inherit a prolapsing mitral valve also inherit a sensitivity of the autonomic nervous system and the tendency for it to go out of balance (Frederickson 1992). This is known as *dysautonomia*, which is pronounced dis-auto-no-me-a. Dysautonomia describes a delayed, inappropriate, or exaggerated response of the autonomic nervous system to a stimulus that can be either internal or external.

An example of a *delayed response* of the autonomic nervous system occurs when you push yourself too hard. For instance, if you spend an entire morning moving furniture and lifting boxes, you may feel perfectly fine the rest of the day. However, by nighttime you may begin experiencing chest pains. The chest pains are a delayed result of the moving and lifting you did, even though you may have done that twelve hours earlier.

Your ANS may respond in an *inappropriate* manner after you have been inside a sauna. For example, the humidity inside a sauna can cause people with dysautonomia to have panic attacks. As a rule, saunas do not cause panic attacks in people without dysautonomia. For this reason, people with dysautonomia should avoid saunas, if possible.

One way your ANS might respond in an *exaggerated* fashion occurs during and after any type of aerobic exercise. For example, while you are exercising, your pulse may rise at an exaggerated rate, or higher than a person's who does not have dysautonomia. It may be several hours before your pulse returns to its normal resting rate. Whereas, the pulse rate of a person without dysautonomia may return to normal within a matter of minutes after exercising.

Your Autonomic Nervous System

The nervous system is composed of several parts, including two systems or sets of "action" nerves. One of these is the voluntary nervous system, the nerves of which conduct the business of such familiar motor tasks as controlling your arm and leg motions. Involuntary, or automatic, functions are governed by a separate system of nerves. These nerves that function automatically (that is, without conscious instructions) are called the autonomic nervous system. The *autonomic nervous system* (ANS) also consists of two sets of components, the *sympathetic* and the *parasympathetic* systems.

The Sympathetic Nervous System and the Parasympathetic Nervous System

The sympathetic nervous system controls many functions, including the rate at which your heartbeat accelerates, your blood pressure increases, and your blood flow decreases. The sympathetic system can be thought of and referred to as the *accelerator* of your nervous system because it prepares your body for stressful situations and emergencies.

For example, imagine that a rabid dog is chasing you down the street and you are running as fast as you can to escape the huge, snarling animal whose mouth is frothing with foam and whose teeth are snapping at your heels. In such a dire situation, your sympathetic nervous system will increase the rate at which you breathe, the rate at which your heart pumps blood, and it also raises your blood pressure. Furthermore, it will redirect blood flow to various organs in your body to help you to react to this danger—so that you can run as fast as you can, as efficiently as your body and the physical condition you are in will permit.

The parasympathetic system controls the opposing effects, that is, it increases blood flow to your muscles and decreases blood pressure, heart rate, and breathing rate. This system can be thought of as the *brakes* of the entire nervous system because it returns the body to its normal state after a stressful situation has ended.

Depending on the needs of your particular body and the amount of stress to which it is subjected, your autonomic nervous system adjusts your body's functions to meet your particular needs. *Any* imbalance in this process can lead to most of the symptoms of dysautonomia.

Neurotransmitters

The sympathetic and parasympathetic nervous systems are constantly monitored by specialized centers in the brain. When the sympathetic system is activated, it releases a neurotransmitter, norepinephrine, from nerve endings, and a hormone, adrenaline, from the adrenal gland.

Activation of the parasympathetic system releases a neurotransmitter from nerve endings called acetylcholine. Put as simply as possible, sympathetic nervous system stimulation usually causes excitatory activity throughout the entire body, while parasympathetic activity serves a more inhibitory function and slows down the excitatory activity.

Most people who have dysautonomia exhibit an excessive degree of sympathetic nervous system activity (Sawyer 1991). Signs of such excessive activity are as follows:

Signs of Excessive Sympathetic Nervous System Activity

- Rapid, strong, or extra heartbeat

- Slow digestion (frequent constipation)

- Alert wakefulness at inappropriate times (sleep difficulties)

- Dilated pupils

Does this collection of symptoms sound familiar to you?

Laura's Story

Laura, who is thirty years old, gets up every morning still tired, even though she goes to bed at 9:00 P.M., because she wakes up wide awake, two or three times every night. It takes her anywhere from half an hour to two hours to fall back asleep again. So, she never really gets a good night's rest. She drags herself out of bed to give her family breakfast and get her kids ready for school, and then she slowly dresses herself and goes to work, wishing she could crawl back into bed and sleep for another two or three hours.

At work, her coworkers find her entertaining because she talks really fast and is very "hyper," and she is a very productive worker. They don't realize that she's constantly worrying about every little thing all day long. By the time Laura arrives home, she is exhausted. Her adrenaline keeps her going well enough to prepare the family's dinner and put the kids to bed. But when she's done with all of the day's tasks, she is so relieved that she cannot wait to climb into bed.

Sleep is hard to come by because Laura has suffered from insomnia for years. It seems her brain simply will not turn off at night, so she lies there and thinks about all of her problems and generally reviews all the negative thoughts running through her mind over and over. She finally gets a couple of hours' sleep before she wakes again, and again, but, of course, after such a night, she is still tired when she rises, and this troubling cycle begins all over again.

If Laura's behavior seems familiar to you, the sympathetic component of your autonomic nervous system may be out of balance. There may be too much excitatory activity going on within you. You may personify the phrase, "Wired and tired."

A small percentage of people with dysautonomia exhibit a demonstrable imbalance of the parasympathetic component of their autonomic nervous system (Sawyer 1991). Signs of this type of imbalance are as follows:

Signs of Imbalance in the Parasympathetic Nervous System

- Slow heart rate

- Abnormally fast digestion (frequent diarrhea)

- Promotes sleep

- Constricted pupils

Gene's Story

Gene, who is also thirty years old, appears to be a laid-back kind of a guy. He goes about his tasks very patiently and methodically. When he has to wait in a long line at the bank, it doesn't bother him at all. If people who don't know him well were to describe him by his outward appearance, they might say he is "calm, cool, and collected."

They would be surprised to learn that Gene knows exactly where every hospital on his way to work is located, just in case he has another panic attack. When he has a panic attack, he thinks he is having a heart attack and he needs to go to the emergency room for help. He also knows where every public restroom on his way to work is located because he suffers from frequent severe bouts of diarrhea. Gene refers to himself as a "laid-back neurotic." He doesn't realize that the parasympathetic component of his autonomic nervous system is out of balance.

Note, too, that there are some people who have *mixed dysautonomia*; that is, they have imbalances in both their sympathetic and parasympathetic nervous systems. What this means is that the biochemical agents, the neurotransmitters and hormones, either exceed the body's needs and/or they fall short of meeting the body's needs. Both of these processes can take place simultaneously, thus causing mixed dysautonomia.

Do You Have Mitral Valve Prolapse (MVP), Dysautonomia, or Both?

Of the two conditions, mitral valve prolapse is definitely easier to diagnose than dysautonomia is. The tests most often used to detect mitral valve prolapse are echocardiograms and stethoscope examinations (see chapter 1). It is also important for your physician to take a complete history of your medical symptoms, together with a complete physical examination, in order to make a proper diagnosis.

Dysautonomia and Doctor Watkins' Theories

Health writer Mary Roach described in very informative detail how she found out that she had dysautonomia in a 1998 article that appeared in *Health Magazine*. In 1983 she had been told there was something wrong with her heart. But it wasn't until she met cardiologist Phillip Watkins, who runs the Mitral Valve Prolapse Center in Birmingham, Alabama, that she discovered, in fact, there was nothing wrong with her heart. She wrote that Dr. Watkins told her that a "floppy" mitral valve is just a "red herring."

He also said that he believes a floppy valve is another symptom of dysautonomia in the nervous system. This dysautonomia results in a very low blood volume, which means that "the body has 80-to-85 percent of the fluid it is supposed to have." Such a low blood volume leads, in turn, to the symptoms of "dizziness, heartbeat irregularities, chest pain, panic attacks, and, most commonly, fatigue. It's like being in a [permanent] state of chronic dehydration." *All* of these symptoms are common among people who have MVPS/D.

When Dr. Watkins examined Ms. Roach, he checked out her hands to see if they were cold. They were. According to Ms. Roach, her hands and her feet were almost always cold. He also asked her the following set of questions:

- "Do you ever get light-headed when you stand up?"

- She answered, "Sometimes."

- He asked, Do you ever have "dry eyes?"

- She said, "Constantly."

- His final question was, "Do you feel run down, and are you easily fatigued?"

- Her simple response, "Yup," led to his diagnosis, which he stated in one short sentence, "Your fluid is low."

Of course Ms. Roach did not understand what he meant by "Your fluid is low." So she questioned him further and he said this:

"If you take a patient with [a] prolapse, turn her upside down, dump out all the fluid from her arteries and veins, it's only about 80 percent of what it should be." He then told Ms. Roach, "You're down by almost a quart." He theorized that a faulty feedback mechanism in the brain fails to signal the body that it needs more water, and said, "It [the body] thinks the tank is full when it isn't."

Dr. Watkins also used other metaphors to describe dysautonomia. He said that you can think of someone with low blood fluid as being like a water balloon that is only partially filled. If you stand that person on end, the fluid, following the law of gravity, will flow down to the lower half of the body, "unlike a fully plumped water balloon, wherein the water stays put." When blood is pooling in the legs, the head doesn't quite get an adequate supply. Because of that, when the person stands up suddenly from a sitting or lying down position, she or he will become light-headed.

Furthermore, low blood volume causes the brain to move blood away from the rest of the body and into the legs. This results in cold hands and feet.

When fluid levels drop, the brain calls upon adrenaline to speed up the rate at which the heart beats. "The less blood there is circulating, the faster the body needs to have oxygen, nutrients, and waste shuttled to and from its cells. The end result is that people with low blood volume suffer a chronic excess of adrenaline."

When Mary Roach asked what a low blood volume had to do with her prolapsing mitral valve, Dr. Watkins responded by saying that the heart itself shrinks because of the decrease in blood volume, but the valve does not shrink; it stays the same size and, then, because it is too big for the heart, it "flops" around.

Ms. Roach then listened to her heart with Dr. Watkins' stethoscope while she was standing up, and she heard "a sound that [was] neither lub nor dub, a small muffled sharpness like fingers being snapped inside [her] chest." That sound was produced by her loose mitral valve.

Then, Dr. Watkins had Ms. Roach lie down on the examining table and she listened to her heart again with his stethoscope. She wrote, "With the blood in my body more evenly distributed, the click is gone." He asked her if her heart ever races for no obvious reason and whether she has panic attacks. Fortunately for Ms. Roach, she does not experience either symptom; but many of Dr. Watkins' patients do exhibit both panic attacks and racing hearts. He believes that both of these symptoms are also caused by low blood volume and the resultant rise in adrenaline.

Al Davies, an endocrinologist from the Baylor College of Medicine in Houston has provided further evidence for this theory. He states:

> Since in MVPS/D, the main problem is oversensitivity to adrenaline, therapy is directed at minimizing releasing adrenaline into the blood, and blocking its actions once it gets there. This means that some adjustments in lifestyle become necessary for most people. A person might notice specific events that seem to trigger the symptoms, so those triggers should be avoided. Therapy may start with a natural way of keeping adrenaline to a minimum—by increasing blood volume with salt (Davies 1996).

Davies has found biochemical evidence that people with dysautonomia not only demonstrate excessive amounts of adrenaline, they are also extremely sensitive to it. He believes that, even if they produced only a normal amount of adrenaline, it would still have a stronger effect on them, which may explain why people with MVPS/D feel so fatigued so much of the time. Ninety-two percent of Dr. Watkins' patients report that they lack energy most of the time (Roach 1998).

Diagnosing Dysautonomia

The best way to determine whether or not you have dysautonomia is by taking the aptly named tilt-table test. The test involves placing you on a table with a foot support. (The foot support is there for you to stand on when the table is tilted 45 or more degrees.) Then the table is tilted upward. The table usually starts the test in a horizontal position and then is gradually tilted upward by degrees to a vertical position. For instance, the table will tilt you up to a 30-degree angle.

Lying at a 30-degree angle feels as though you're lying on a steep hill. You are tilted upright so that your head is always above your feet. You are never turned upside down. Your blood pressure and electrocardiogram (EKG) will be checked for several minutes while you are in this position. Then, the table will tilt your body up to a 60-degree angle.

Even when you are lying on a table that is tilted at a 60-degree angle, it feels as though you are standing on the footboard at the bottom of the table. You are still weight-bearing. When you take this test you will have two safety straps placed around your waist and your knees to make you feel more secure. At the 60-degree angle, your heart rate is evaluated again. That is done because changes in heart rate combined with the changes in posture reflect how well your autonomic nervous system is functioning.

While you are positioned on the tilt table other simple tests will be performed. These tests also reflect the functioning of your autonomic nervous system. For example, you will be asked to perform the Valsalva maneuver by trying to forcibly exhale for fifteen seconds with your nose, mouth, and glottis closed. It is like blowing up a balloon. Still lying on the table, you will also take a handgrip test, while your blood pressure and heart rate changes are recorded. Your blood pressure and cardiac output (the amount of blood the heart actually pumps out) are also evaluated.

What the Tilt-Table Test Shows

Tilt-table testing is designed to evaluate how your autonomic nervous system regulates blood pressure in response to some very simple stresses. If the nerves in your autonomic nervous system that control blood pressure are not operating properly, they may have a reaction that causes your blood pressure to drop suddenly. This reaction can produce a number of the symptoms of dysautonomia, including severe light-headedness. Tilt-table testing is designed to determine the likelihood that you are susceptible to this type of reaction, and thus, whether or not you have dysautonomia.

With the results of this test a determination is made as to the nature of the imbalance of your autonomic nervous system. Then, treatment appropriate for your particular type of imbalance can be chosen. Note that you may be retested later to evaluate your progress. Remember, one can have mitral valve prolapse with dysautonomia and mitral valve prolapse without dysautonomia, but quite often they occur together.

Not every hospital has the facilities or trained personnel to perform tilt-table testing. Furthermore, if you do find a hospital to give you the test, your health insurance may not pay for it. So, what can you do in such a case? Fortunately, there is a less expensive, relatively easy-to-administer and easy-to-take test called the Prolonged Standing Test that also can determine dysautonomia. Your family physician can perform this test.

To obtain the most accurate results, your physician will have you lie down for several minutes. Then, you stand up, and your blood pressure and heart rate will be measured at one-minute intervals for three to five minutes. Depending on the rates at which your blood pressure and heart rate rise or fall, your physician should be able to determine whether dysautonomia is likely to be present.

What if your echocardiogram is negative, a tilt-table test is not available, and you can't have a prolonged standing test performed? Unfortunately, there are physicians who either do not believe in mitral valve prolapse syndrome and/or dysautonomia, or who do not understand this disorder, and are very reluctant to take the time to give patients a prolonged standing test.

If you still feel that you have dysautonomia, you must try to find a physician who is open-minded, compassionate, and willing to take the time to talk with you. As Dr. Watkins once remarked, "We should treat the patients, not their ECHO tests. If it walks like a duck, talks like a duck, and looks like a duck, you'll probably get it to quack for you."

Personal Reflections on Dysautonomia

The following stories are provided so that you will have some clinical information against which to compare your own symptoms. These reflections are also included here because they offer you hope. You are not alone, and you are not losing your mind. It is our belief that these stories will provide you with details that will illuminate your own physical experiences. We also hope that if these stories do speak to you because they resemble your own experiences, that you will take them to heart and seek both a proper diagnosis and proper treatment for dysautonomia. Note that the identities of all of the writers have been disguised to protect their privacy.

Nancy's Story

"In July of 1996, I was sitting in yet another doctor's office. This time the visit was to a cardiologist to see if perhaps he could identify the reason for my perpetual shortness of breath, my irregular heartbeat, and my hypersensitivity to any form of physical exertion. He listened to my symptoms, examined my twenty-year-old body, noted my tiny frame, long fingers, and straight back. He read the meticulous outline of topics (more than a little obsessively researched) that I had organized for our discussion, including my personal suggestions for possible tests, diagnosis, and medications. Within five minutes, even before doing an echocardiogram, he said that he was almost positive that he knew what I had: mitral valve prolapse and the accompanying syndrome.

"It all fit perfectly; from my family history of MVP, to my problems with a panic/anxiety disorder since the age of fourteen, my highly driven personality and need for perfectionism, even to my physical appearance, and all the physical complaints I described. Sure enough, the ECHO test revealed mitral valve prolapse. The doctor explained that the severity of my symptoms was not related to the severity of the prolapse. I happen to have a relatively mild case of prolapse, but my dysautonomic symptoms at times make my life almost unbearable.

"My symptoms have tended to be cardiovascular in nature. I have a racing heart, for which I have taken a beta-blocker for five years (the relief this has provided for me is indescribable), and pre-atrial contractions. Sometimes my heart 'skips' about every third beat for days at a time, and I suffer from shortness of breath. Stress aggravates my problems enormously. For example, if I take a difficult exam at school, I can count on experiencing one or more symptoms in the following days.

"My most debilitating symptom, however, is one that no doctor I've ever visited has even heard of; it is the shortness of breath I experience every single morning. After waking, I have to wait at least two to three hours before I can do any physical activity, even something as easy as walking to campus. This is how long it takes my body to adjust in the morning each and every day. Whenever I try to perform any physical task before the morning has passed, I nearly pass out, and I wind up with the sensation of being out of breath for as long as a week's duration. I am continuing to search for a way to ease this problem.

"Over the course of seven years I have consulted countless general practitioners, a cardiologist, an ear, nose, and throat doctor (for help dealing with several months of unexplained dizziness), a psychologist, emergency room doctors (for a spell of irregular heartbeats that really scared me during my sophomore year at college), an endocrinologist (my catecholamines can run high, but not high enough to indicate any glandular disorder), a pediatric nephrologist, and even a sleep specialist. I have had more medical tests performed on me than anyone else I know. When test results come back in the normal range every time, it's both good and bad news. I need to know why my body does the bizarre things it does. I don't want to be told that these symptoms are 'all in my head.' Mitral valve prolapse syndrome is the first diagnosis I've ever received that makes any kind of sense.

"Some of the doctors I've seen were so condescending that I wanted to punch them out. But I've also had doctors who took me seriously and respected my concerns. My primary care physician and my cardiologist are two of the latter, and they have provided me with excellent care."

Nancy's story is fairly typical of a person with dysautonomia. It would seem that a large number of people who have MVPS/D must visit several physicians before being properly diagnosed. Also, it is not surprising that Nancy feels that some doctors were very condescending toward her. Unfortunately, there are doctors who either don't know there is a syndrome that accompanies mitral valve prolapse, or they simply don't believe that such a syndrome exists.

Chris's Story

"Hi, my name is Chris. I am twenty-six years old and the mother of two-year-old twins. I was first diagnosed with mitral valve prolapse in late 1993, a few months after getting married. My symptoms were chest pains and spells when breathing became difficult. After seeing several doctors, and receiving no answers, let alone a name for my problem, it was a relief when I finally got the diagnosis.

"It seemed then that knowing what I had and that it was not life-threatening was enough to keep it under control. In fact, for quite a while, I was rarely bothered by mitral valve prolapse. But all of the symptoms I had previously had plus a bunch of others reared their ugly heads again eight months ago, immediately after we moved from an apartment to a house. I have been suffering now since last April with the chest pains and shortness of breath, as well as with panic attacks, enormous feelings of anxiety, fatigue, a racing heartbeat, dizziness, and nausea.

"I sought help immediately from a new doctor, since we no longer lived near the old one. He told me I was just suffering from anxiety. Of course, tell me, who wouldn't be anxious with two young children and having just moved into a new house? From then until now I have simply lived with these conditions. I was convinced, bottom line, that I needed to relax. I tried, and tried, and tried. Sometimes things seemed better, but often, they were worse. But I lived with it and sought no other help. For a long time 'denial' got me through.

"During the past month or so I decided there must be something else wrong with me. Brain tumor? Cancer? Or had my mitral valve prolapse gone really bad? Every aspect of my life has been suffering. I am short-tempered with my children. I was a long-distance runner for more than ten years, but I haven't been enjoying it for months because of my speeded-up heart rate and my problems with breathing. Nighttime is the worst; I have begun to feel afraid of the dark. Not that the bogeyman is going to get me, but that I am being enveloped by the darkness.

"Last night was a typical experience for me, lately. I went to bed around 11:00 P.M. and drifted off to sleep pretty easily (although often I lie awake and think of all the awful things that could happen to my family). At 12:30, my daughter cried out to me, so I got up, put her in our bed, and went downstairs to the bathroom. When I returned to bed and tried to go back to sleep my heart began to race, my chest hurt, I was nauseated, and I began obsessing about terrible thoughts. I tossed and turned and knew that, soon, I would either be dead of a fatal disease, or institutionalized because I had finally gone crazy. My husband woke up about an hour later, after I had put our daughter back in her own bed. We talked a bit, and finally sleep found me.

"Today, I made an appointment with another cardiologist. I cried a lot and yelled at my children far too much. A few hours ago, my husband called and insisted that I should visit him at his workplace. He just got a new computer and now can get on the Internet. He wanted to see whether I could find some information on the Net that might help me. He took the kids away for an hour, and I searched. That's when it happened, and here I sit, both excited and more relieved than I have been in a very, very long time. I stumbled on The Mitral Valve Prolapse Society and all its information.

"I sat there reading and wanted to cry. I felt like I was reading all about myself. I never knew anything about mitral valve prolapse in such depth. I thought it would only affect, or should I say cause, breathing problems, chest pains, and irregular heartbeats. An 'out-of-balance' nervous system! That's what I have. I am not going crazy! I do not have a brain tumor or cancer! My anxiety and panic attacks can be explained. For the first time in a long time I feel hope that I can return to living a normal life.

"Well, I won't go on, though I easily could. I just felt compelled to share my story and to make people aware of the difference this new information I have discovered has already made in my life."

It is terrifying to try to go about your daily routine, and live a normal life, all the while thinking that you might be suffering from a terminal illness, or that you are "going crazy." Obviously, it brought tremendous relief to Chris when she found out that she has MVPS/D. Equally important was her discovery that her illness has a name, and that others have it, too. This gave her the hope she will need to learn how to cope with her symptoms, and return to living a normal life.

Frank's Story

"I am a thirty-seven-year-old man. I was diagnosed with MVP in the beginning of 1996. The day it happened, my heart took off out of control, and my whole chest cavity was shaking. Of course, when we finally got to the emergency room, the shaking had stopped. But the speed at which my heart was racing was still 150, then 138, and then 120 for a while, until it slowed to normal. [Editor's note: a normal heart beats at 50 to 100 beats per minute.] They said they couldn't find anything wrong and they sent me home. They said it was a freak occurrence, and not to worry about it. That was easy enough for them to say.

"My next appointment was with my father's cardiologist. He listened and said he had 'heard a click.' He also said, 'Don't worry. It's probably nothing,' but he instructed me to do nothing until I had a stress test. Okay, it's freak-out time! I'm thirty-three years old, married to a woman seven years my junior. We have a ten-month old child, and I'm thinking I'm going to die!

"Mind you, I always worked like a dog, smoked, was a caffeine freak, and drank like a fish. I was also about twenty pounds overweight, but I never had a health problem until then, and I was scared to death.

"Well, I aced the stress test and then I had an echocardiogram. The results were mitral valve prolapse. No problem, lots of people have it. But stop smoking and drinking caffeine and beer. Thank God I married a nurse. God does work in mysterious ways. I own my own company, and I always lived with heavy-duty stress, and now no beer and cigarettes. I quit cold turkey, just like that. I wanted to live. I exercised, ate right, and I went to bed early. I actually exercised myself sick. I dropped from 205 to 155 pounds, and my blood sugar was being depleted because my metabolism had changed. The doctor said just to do cardiovascular exercise a few times a week and eat more. Now I'm a healthy 173 pounds.

"Then it happened! I was at the Atlanta Olympics watching a basketball game, and I had a panic attack. I had another in my car going to my office. I had panic attacks three times on my way to the emergency room. I felt like a real nut case. My whole family was worried about me, and I had another daughter on the way. I thought I was going to die. I saw a doctor about hypoglycemia who told me that I was fine, but a nervous wreck. He sent me to a friend of his who was a shrink. A shrink. I didn't need a shrink. But I knew something was wrong. I figured maybe it was an old head injury from my motorcycle accident, or maybe it was because of the time a golf ball hit me in the head, so I went to a neurologist. He had me take an MRI and a brain wave test. Everything was normal. So, I gave in and saw the shrink.

"I told him that nowadays I hate driving, and I hate big buildings that I used to love to go to for sporting events, and that a couple of times a week I have panic attacks. After four visits, he told me I was the sanest person he had met in a long time. He also said, 'You have great willpower, but I would bet that you have mitral valve prolapse syndrome.' He put me on an anti-anxiety medication, which did the trick. I hate the medication and I would love a beer, but I guess that's life. You win some and you lose some.

"Some of the other symptoms I have include cold hands and feet and a slow heart rate. I also have some jaw pain, and, recently, chest pain that was so bad it scared the hell out of me. The doctor thinks it's skeletal. I also get cold sweats and I sometimes have dizzy spells.

"But I have been relatively okay. I think the worst part of this condition is the syndrome—not the mitral valve prolapse itself. The syndrome is not well-known, and I went through a terrible time of thinking that I was going crazy. It's a very humbling experience.

Also, it took altogether too long to get the right medications. I still go into large sporting centers and malls very slowly, very cautiously. I hate them. I was never like that before until the day that I had so many panic attacks. It was like my whole system was switched from 'normal' to 'off.'

"I think it is wonderful that I finally found some information about mitral valve prolapse syndrome and dysautonomia, and I hope my story helps someone else. I still go to events, ride Harleys, and, fortunately, I have good stamina, so far. The secret to living with this syndrome, I guess, is a combination of the right medications, exercise, support from your family, and a sense of humor."

Frank is correct about the keys to coping with MVPS/D. Along with exercising, eating right, and other lifestyle modifications, it is extremely important to surround yourself with supportive people. Also, for those days when you're just not feeling "up to par," there is nothing like a well-developed sense of humor to keep you going.

If you have MVPS/D, you should be able to relate to these very personal stories. It can be extremely helpful when you know that other people have gone through what you are experiencing and to find out what their coping mechanisms are. These stories demonstrate that you are not the only one to experience this set of symptoms. You are not alone, and you are not going crazy! Remember, although the stories may seem very similar, no two people exhibit exactly the same set of symptoms, or the same severity of symptoms.

CHAPTER 3

The Physical Symptoms of Mitral Valve Prolapse/Dysautonomia

A wise man should consider that health is the greatest of human blessings and learn how by his own thought to derive benefit from his illness.

—Hippocrates

If you have mitral valve prolapse syndrome/dysautonomia (MVPS/D), you may experience an array of troublesome and often frightening symptoms. These symptoms can affect your lifestyle and the way you go about your daily routines and living your life. For example, if you're always terribly fatigued, you won't be able to accomplish everything you need to do in one day. What others would accomplish in one day might take you three or four days— even a week. If you have severe irritable bowel syndrome, you may need to curtail your movements and put limits on where you can go in order to be close to a bathroom just in case you need one.

Common Symptoms of MVPS/D

The good news is that the symptoms of MVPS/D either can be eased or remedied by implementing certain techniques and/or lifestyle changes. The main idea behind these techniques or lifestyle changes is to correct your autonomic nervous system gently to get it to move back into balance.

Fatigue

Fatigue is one of the most common symptoms of MVPS/D. This fatigue is not caused by becoming tired or weary, as everyone does from time to time at the end of the day. This is an overwhelming lack of energy that is present most of the time. Fatigue caused by MVPS/D can turn a seemingly simple task, like vacuuming the living room carpet, into a major chore (see chapter 8).

The issue that adds extra stress to your life and can make matters immeasurably worse is that the people closest to you do not understand the nature of your problem. Mitral valve prolapse syndrome/dysautonomia is invisible, and many people may not understand exactly how fatigued you can become. They may imply that you are lazy, spoiled, selfish, or that you are malingering to get out of your responsibilities. Or they may think that you are just plain crazy. Even those people with MVPS/D who suffer from only mild fatigue may become frustrated at not having as much energy as they used to have.

For example, when Karen was raising her three small children, she rushed through every afternoon to prepare the family's dinner as early as it was possible to do. It took her years to realize that the reason that she rushed that way was the overwhelming fatigue she experienced in the middle of the afternoon. Her fatigue was so severe that all she wanted to do was get dinner on the table and over with, wash and put the dishes away, and lie down and rest.

For most people with MVPS/D, there usually is a particular time of the day when the fatigue caused by the syndrome is at its worst, making you feel as though all the energy has been drained from your body. The most common time for this to occur is in the late afternoon. But everyone has a different body, and you may feel the most fatigue early in the morning, the early afternoon, or the early evening.

Many of you have probably noticed that when you overexert yourself for a couple of days in a row, by the third day, your fatigue is so bad, you feel as though you've been run over by a truck. At other times, there may be no apparent reason for the fatigue you experience. Oftentimes, fatigue results from being out of shape; however, this is not always the case. The vast majority of people with MVPS/D have low blood pressure and low blood volume, both of which contribute to fatigue. Other causes of fatigue are lack of the proper amount of restful sleep, a diet high in sugar and caffeine, and overexertion.

Exercise

Exercise is the key to alleviating fatigue and, in fact, it is probably the most important component in treating dysautonomia. When you are first beginning an exercise program, you may find yourself even more fatigued than usual, until you build up to your optimal strength level. Unless you have other problems, such as arthritis, that level should be at least thirty minutes of aerobic activity at least three days a week (see chapter 11).

You also need to limit your sugar intake and, if possible, eliminate caffeine. Note that eating high-protein snacks in the morning and afternoon may boost your energy level.

Heart Palpitations

When you have heart palpitations, they can make you feel as though your heart is not beating properly. Note that whether you describe the palpitations as "flutters," "flip-flops," or "skipped heartbeats," they all fall into the category of palpitations.

Frequently, when people feel palpitations, they think they are having heart attacks and they go to the nearest emergency room. However, there are quite a number of causes for such palpitations, including overexertion, fatigue, illness, PMS, menopause, stress, stimulants, alcohol, panic attacks, tobacco, lifting heavy weights, and lying on your left side.

Regardless of what causes these palpitations, experiencing them may cause anxiety. Those that are caused by MVPS/D are harmless, as opposed to other types of palpitations caused by heart disease. Remember, people with MVPS/D and/or structural mitral valve prolapse have normal, functioning hearts.

To control palpitations it is extremely important to keep yourself well hydrated and to eliminate stimulants and alcohol from your diet. Obviously, you should stop smoking, as that is detrimental in any number of ways. In addition, a very low dosage of a beta-blocker may eliminate palpitations. Note that, while experiencing palpitations, many people feel an urge to cough. Believe it or not, coughing one or two times is very likely to stop the palpitations.

Bear in mind that palpitations of the heart are among the most frightening physical experiences that people can have. They can be especially frightening to those with MVPS/D, because such people naturally have increased levels of cardiac awareness. They may be conscious of every heartbeat and, furthermore, they may perceive their hearts as pounding or beating more forcefully than they really are.

This hyperawareness can be present even when people with MVPS/D demonstrate a fairly normal pulse rate. Many of those with this syndrome describe their feelings of cardiac awareness as someone might describe his or her cardiac behavior after vigorous exercise; but those with MVPS/D experience such awareness at rest, lying down, or while trying to fall asleep.

Often exhaustive cardiac testing will be done to reassure you that there is nothing seriously wrong with your heart. Therefore, at those times that you do experience symptoms such as palpitations, these symptoms should become more tolerable to you after cardiac testing, because you will have the peace of mind of knowing that your heart is okay.

Premature Ventricular Contractions

Premature ventricular contractions (PVCs) are one of the minor arrhythmias that affect many people, but especially those with MVPS/D. They are often observed in the EKGs of adults, with or without MVPS/D, monitored over a period of hours.

The *Merck Manual* describes PVCs as extra heartbeats caused by electrical activation of the ventricles before the normal heartbeat. Premature ventricular contractions are fairly common, and they don't indicate any danger for those who do not have underlying heart disease.

Many people have PVCs and don't even know it. Because people with MVPS/D are more aware of their heartbeat they tend to feel PVCs quite clearly. The main symptom people complain of is a strong or skipped beat. These PVCs have little effect on the pumping action of the heart.

Recommendations for treatment include reducing stress and avoiding alcohol and over-the-counter cold medicines containing stimulants.

Tachycardia

Tachycardia is the name for a rapid or speeded-up heart rate. You may experience this even when you have not exerted yourself at all. That is because your autonomic nervous system "thinks" that you are doing something much more strenuous than you actually are. For example, when Dan, who does *not* have MVPS/D, climbs a flight of stairs, he has an increased heart rate of ten to twelve beats.

When Carol, who *does* have MVPS/D, climbs the same flight of stairs, her heart rate increases by forty beats, or more.

Tachycardia often keeps people from continuing with their exercise programs, because they think they're going to have a heart attack. This is doubly unfortunate because exercising regularly is one way to alleviate tachycardia. Another way is to eliminate caffeine from your diet, as much as is possible.

Headaches

Research undertaken by the University of California at San Diego found that men and women with MVPS/D have a greater tendency to suffer from headaches than the normal population (Ford and Ford 1996).

Types of Headaches

Several types of headaches can be caused by MVPS/D. The most common are *tension headaches*. This is, typically, a steady, dull ache, rather than a throbbing one, and it affects both sides of the head. It may also be chronic, occurring frequently, or even daily.

Cluster headaches are relatively rare and affect mostly men and boys. These are headaches that come in groups, or clusters, that last for weeks or even for months. The pain is extreme, but the headache, fortunately, is brief, often lasting not more than one or two hours.

Classical migraines are less common than tension headaches, but they are one of the basic types of headaches associated with MVPS/D (Cotton 1992). They are far more prevalent among women than men. Roughly three out of four migraine sufferers are female.

Most people feel migraines only on one side of their head, and the pain is, typically, throbbing in nature. Nausea, with or without vomiting, and extreme sensitivity to light and sound, often accompany migraines. Sometimes, an aura, or a group of telltale neuralgic symptoms, is experienced before the head pain begins. About one in five migraine attacks occur only occasionally, but sometimes they are as frequent as once or twice a week. They rarely occur daily.

There is also a condition known as *migraine equivalent*. This occurs when you have the equivalent of a migraine without the pain, but the aura is present. Sometimes, when this occurs you also may notice the hair on your arms standing up. Migraine equivalent appears to be very common among people with MVPS/D.

Headache Triggers

There are various triggers thought to activate the processes that cause headaches in those who are prone to them. If you suffer from headaches, we recommend keeping a headache diary to help you identify those factors in your life that trigger your headaches.

Common Headache Triggers

- Skipping meals, especially breakfast; and/or fasting

- Eating chocolate, processed meats (containing nitrates), aged cheese, MSG; drinking too much caffeine or red wine

- Taking nitroglycerin

- Napping, oversleeping, or getting too little sleep

- Feeling extreme heat or cold, high humidity, windy conditions

- Experiencing bright lights, office lighting, flashing lights, or odors, pollution, smog, perfumes, and/or chemicals

- Experiencing estrogen level changes, menstruation, side effects from hormone replacement therapies, birth control pill changes

There are measures you can take to prevent migraines. These include maintaining regular sleep patterns, exercising regularly, eating well-balanced meals at the same time of day every day, and reducing the stress in your life as much as possible. Biofeedback, a technique where you learn how to control some of your body's internal functions, can be useful for preventing headaches. Relaxation training, stress management, hypnosis, and acupuncture are also helpful. There are several over-the-counter medications that treat headaches. If these don't work, consult your physician, because there are many prescription medications specifically for headaches.

Note that some medications for migraines contain large amounts of caffeine. You actually may have to choose between the effects of the caffeine or getting rid of your headache.

For example, Judy occasionally gets migraine headaches. She also has tachycardia. She has to decide whether she should take the over-the-counter medication that she knows will rid her of her headache while at the same time worsening her tachycardia because of its high caffeine content. If she has to go to work that day, Judy usually takes the medication and tolerates the tachycardia.

Irritable Bowel Syndrome

The primary symptoms of irritable bowel syndrome (IBS) include abdominal pain, diarrhea, and constipation. These vary greatly in frequency and intensity. Other common symptoms are indigestion, nausea, gas, and bloating. Although IBS can be devastating for the sufferer, it actually feels worse than it is. Fortunately, it does not make you more susceptible to other bowel diseases or cancer.

Although many times IBS attacks occur out of the blue, alcohol and caffeine can trigger them. A diet high in fiber is one way to keep the condition under control, whether your symptoms are diarrhea or constipation.

Irritable bowel syndrome is also associated with lactose intolerance, which is a sensitivity to dairy products. Exercise and stress reduction help to lessen bouts of IBS. Since most people with MVPS/D have a low blood volume, it is extremely important for them to replenish their fluids after undergoing a bout of diarrhea.

Gastroesophageal Reflux Disease

Gastroesophageal reflux disease (GERD) is a fairly common problem for people with MVPS/D, especially for those who also have IBS. This is a condition in which acid from the stomach flows backward up into the esophagus. It can cause chest pain and a sensation of discomfort that feels like burning. The pain may radiate to the neck and arms. Sometimes, the acid moves up toward the throat and causes a bitter or acid taste.

The burning and pressure symptoms of heartburn can last for several hours and they often worsen after eating. The pain is similar to angina or heart problems. For these reasons, GERD causes much concern, and people often seek help for it by going to the emergency room.

Treatment can be as simple as lifestyle modifications, including avoiding foods and beverages like chocolate, coffee, peppermint, greasy or spicy foods, tomato products, and alcohol. If you smoke, stop. Tobacco may stimulate acid production. Do not eat two or three hours before bedtime. Overeating and excess weight can contribute to reflux.

If you suffer from GERD try elevating the head of your bed six to eight inches. For infrequent episodes of heartburn try an over-the-counter antacid. For GERD that doesn't respond to antacids, see your physician. Many new prescription medications are available to help this problem.

Chest Pain

Chest pain is another frightening symptom. Along with panic attacks and heart palpitations, chest pain is one of the main reasons people rush to the emergency room of the nearest hospital. Many people feel a sharp pain in their chests, while others feel more of a burning or sticking, stabbing feeling.

Some people always feel their pain in the same location, such as in the middle of their chest, while others feel it in different locations each time it occurs. It may be on your left side one month and your right side the next month. You can also have pain in your armpit or pain that starts in your chest and radiates through your back.

There are several ways to deal with chest pain. One is to exercise regularly. For many people, elevating their feet when they begin to feel chest pain works well. Michelle often watches TV from the floor of her bedroom with her legs high up on her bed, so as to prevent chest pain.

Fluid loading is also very important. You should drink a minimum of eight glasses of eight ounces of fluid per day. That's sixty-four ounces of fluid. When it is warmer outside, drink one ounce per each degree of the outside temperature. For example, if it is 80 degrees outside, you should drink eighty ounces of nonalcoholic fluid (see chapter 7).

Sleep Disorders

It seems as though the majority of people with MVPS/D have sleeping problems. Most of the complaints appear to fall into the insomnia category. Typically, you may experience difficulty falling asleep, and once asleep, you frequently awaken, and, basically, you experience disrupted sleep throughout the night. This type of sleep pattern can be a significant contributing factor to your daytime tiredness or fatigue. Unlike many other people with similar sleep disorders, often you may be very conscious or aware of the arousals and awakenings that occur during your sleep and can describe the events quite descriptively, thus indicating that you don't ever fall into a really deep sleep.

Nocturnal myoclonus, or periodic twitching of legs and arms during sleep, is another sleep problem. For example, just when John felt as though he was about to fall asleep, one of his legs would suddenly begin to twitch. His leg would actually kick up into the air several inches, which would wake him, and then he would have to try to fall asleep all over again. There is also a condition called a *nocturnal panic attack*. This causes people to awaken suddenly with tachycardia (an abnormally rapid heartbeat) and a sense of panic.

To promote a more restful sleep, try not to eat heavy meals in the evening. Stay away from stimulants, and do not exercise late in the day. Another good idea is to try to wind down a couple of hours before bedtime. Although you may be exhausted, by the end of the day your mind will not automatically shut down. Therefore, you should avoid such activities as late-night telephone conversations, paying your bills, balancing your checkbook, and so forth. Note that if all else fails, you may be able to find help at a clinic that specializes in sleep disorders (see chapter 8).

Dizziness

Dizziness, lightheadedness, and feeling faint are very common symptoms with MVPS/D. These symptoms are frequently associated with heart fluttering and pounding. They can be exacerbated by heat, humidity, dehydration, and low blood pressure. Although you may feel faint many times, in actuality, fainting spells are extremely rare.

You can greatly decrease episodes of dizziness and lightheadedness by drinking sixty-four ounces of fluid a day, more in the summertime. To retain these fluids, you need to increase your salt intake. Do *not* increase salt intake if you are one of the minority with MVPS/D who also has high blood pressure.

Ways to Lessen Dizziness

- Eat smaller, more frequent meals. Avoid large meals, because blood pressure may become quite low after eating.

- Avoid sugar. It decreases blood pressure.

- Get out of beds or chairs slowly.

- Avoid strenuous activities in hot weather.

- Plan activities for the afternoon. Blood pressure is usually at its lowest in the morning.

- If you have an extreme case of dizziness, there are medications to increase blood pressure. The lower your blood pressure, the greater the chance you have of becoming dizzy or lightheaded.

Fibromyalgia

Many people who have MVPS/D also have fibromyalgia (FM). The symptoms of each are almost identical, and, in fact, some people believe MVPS/D, FM, chronic fatigue syndrome, and perhaps temporomandibular joint dysfunction (TMJ) are most likely one and the same syndrome. If they are not, they may be very closely related.

Although fibromyalgia may feel like a joint disease, it is not a true form of arthritis and does not cause deformities of the joints. Fibromyalgia is characterized by an enhanced sensitivity to pain and by chronic fatigue. It is now believed to be caused by a central nervous system dysfunction (Starlanyl and Copeland 2001).

Pain is the most prominent symptom of fibromyalgia. Although it may start in one region, such as the neck and shoulders, it generally occurs throughout the body and spreads over a period of time. The pain has been described in a variety of ways, including burning, gnawing, soreness, stiffness, and aches. People with FM also experience moderate to severe fatigue. Most people with FM also have an associated sleep disorder.

Other symptoms may include numbness and tingling of hands and feet, headaches, irritable bowel syndrome (IBS), and extreme sensitivity to temperature changes. Eleven sets of tender, sore spots located in specific places throughout the body are the key to a proper diagnosis of fibromyalgia. By the way, have you noticed how similar this condition is to MVPS/D?

Factors That Aggravate Fibromyalgia

- Stressful situations

- Extreme hot or cold weather

- Prolonged sitting or standing

- Moderate physical exertion

Treatment Options for Fibromyalgia

There are many current treatment options including trigger point injections, myofascial release, pain medications, exercise programs, fluid loading, relaxation techniques, and dietary changes. It has been suggested by Regina Gilliland, M.D., that lowering your carbohydrate intake, especially during flare-ups, also may be helpful (Gilliland 1997).

Premenstrual Syndrome

A fairly high percentage of women have premenstrual syndrome (PMS). It is usually characterized by mood swings, feelings of fatigue and depression, headaches, backaches, irritability, bloating, weight gain, and a craving for sweets. These symptoms are felt anywhere from one to two weeks before menstruation and usually stop with the onset of the period. For some women PMS is merely a minor annoyance; for others it is incapacitating.

Some women have found that following an aerobic exercise program reduces symptoms of PMS. Also, be sure to continue to drink a lot of fluids. Many women do not want to load fluids because of the fear of adding to the bloating associated with PMS. But if you exercise, the fluid is dispersed throughout the body as it is needed, instead of collecting in the abdominal wall. Also, consume more vitamins B6 and E, and eliminate caffeine, nicotine, and alcohol from your diet.

Tinnitus

Many people who experience dizziness caused by a dysautonomic disorder will also experience tinnitus, which is the medical name for noises or ringing in the ears. Tinnitus may come and go, or you may be aware of a continuous sound. You may hear it in one or both ears. The sound can vary from a low roar to a high squeal or whine. Although these noises in the ear may, at times, be maddening, they do not affect your hearing.

It is important, however, that you get a thorough exam from your otolaryngologist (ear, nose, and throat specialist) to rule out other problems. Once you receive a diagnosis of tinnitus, you should try to stop worrying about the noise.

A colleague of ours has had constant noise in both ears for the last six years, and he has learned to live with this noise. He says the sound is very similar to the one you hear when you put a seashell up to your ear.

Ways to Lessen the Severity of Tinnitus

- Avoid exposure to loud sounds and noises.

- Avoid stimulants such as coffee, tea, cola, and tobacco.

- Get adequate rest.

- Recognize the noise in your head as an annoyance, and learn to ignore it as much as possible.

- Be sure to ask your physician or pharmacist if any medication you are currently taking might be aggravating your tinnitus. Aspirin and anti-inflammatories are notorious for exacerbating the problem.

In most cases there is no specific treatment for ear and/or head noise. Sometimes, though, concentration and relaxation techniques can reduce the intensity of tinnitus. There is a new technique called masking, which uses a competing sound at a constant low level, like a ticking clock. With masking, the tinnitus may be hidden and, therefore, less noticeable. As of today, one company offers custom-made anti-tinnitus masking CDs (see Resources).

A new FDA-approved device may provide some peace and quiet for people with tinnitus. It is a hand-held probe that is pressed against the mastoid bone behind the ear. Users tune a dial on a separate control unit to a frequency that matches their tinnitus sound, effectively canceling it out (see Resources).

Secondary Symptoms of MVPS/D

- Feeling hot or cold: But these sensations may not be at all related to external temperature. Many people with MVPS/D complain of very cold hands and cold feet regardless of the time of year or of the air temperature.

- Intolerance to heat and the sun: Many people with MVPS/D cannot tolerate being in the sun too long, or in too much heat. Furthermore, high humidity can precipitate panic attacks in such people.

- Shakiness: Sometimes, people with MVPS/D experience shaky hands or legs for no apparent reason.

- Swelling of arms and legs: For someone with MVPS/D, it is usually their feet that have the tendency to swell, especially when that person has been sitting in one position for a long period of time. If you are traveling on an airplane for more than an hour, you should leave your seat and walk up and down the aisle a few times an hour to keep your feet from swelling.

- Shortness of breath: People with MVPS/D are often out of shape because of their low energy levels. This is very much a vicious cycle, because the poorer your condition, the lower your tolerance for any kind of activity. You may notice your heart rate increases greatly with minimal exertion, and you become short of breath. Exercising regularly will alleviate this symptom.

- Numbness in any part of the body: This can happen for absolutely no reason. When it does, your hands and feet feel as if they're "asleep."

- Excessive perspiration or inability to perspire: Suppose two women with MVPS/D are in the same aerobics class, and they do identical sets of exercise for the same length of time. At the end of the session, one woman may be sweating profusely, and the other may look as though she had barely lifted a finger.

- Fibrocystic breast disorder: This is a condition in which a woman may have "lumpy" breasts that become especially tender and sore before menstruation. Avoiding caffeine approximately ten days before menstruation should alleviate some of the tenderness and soreness.

- Skin trouble or rashes: Some people with MVPS/D get hives, eczema, or psoriasis. Over-the-counter creams or gels often help these problems.

- Trouble concentrating or memory problems: Those who have MVPS/D sometimes have days where they can't remember the simplest things, such as a word, a name, and so forth. They also may have trouble concentrating because they sometimes experience the feeling of being "spaced out."

- Heightened sensitivity: MVPS/D may be accompanied by a heightened sense of smell or hearing. For example, it is difficult for some people with the condition to walk past a cosmetic counter because the many scents make them nauseous or give them an immediate headache. If you have a heightened sense of hearing, loud noises such as those made by electric saws and lawn mowers may bother you, and you probably keep the volume on the TV much lower than other people prefer.

- Temporomandibular joint dysfunction (TMJ): In simple terms, this is a misalignment of the jaw. If you have this, your jaw may sometimes make a "clicking" or "popping" noise when you're eating, chewing, yawning, or talking. This symptom also disguises itself as an earache. In fact, many people are diagnosed with TMJ when they visit their doctor for what they think is just an earache. Temporomandibular joint dysfunction can be painful. You may need to use an ice pack, a heating pad, and/or a medication, e.g., ibuprofen to get some relief.

- Scoliosis: This is the name given to curvature of the spine. It is sometimes found in conjunction with MVPS/D. Scoliosis must be diagnosed by a physician.

- Exaggerated startle reflex: If you have this, whenever the telephone rings, you may practically jump out of your chair, even if you were expecting it to ring.

- Low body temperature: A lot of people with MVPS/D have a body temperature lower than the average of 98.6 degrees.

- Endometriosis: This is a disease in which tissue normally found in the uterus is also found in the abdomen, on the ovaries and abdominal lining, and on the bowel and bladder. The most common complaints of this condition are severe and chronic pelvic pain, disabling menstrual periods, repeated miscarriages, painful sexual intercourse, infertility, painful bowel movements, and chronic fatigue. You must see your gynecologist for treatment if you have any of these symptoms.

Other Secondary Symptoms

Mitral valve prolapse syndrome/dysautonomia also may cause any of the following secondary symptoms:

- Nausea

- Neck aches or pain

- Arm and leg aches

- Backaches

- Aches or pains in hands or feet

- Excessive gas

- Hay fever or other allergies

When someone first sees the list of symptoms associated with MVPS/D, that person is often shocked and cannot believe the complexity of the disorder. You may feel the same way. Don't allow this list to overwhelm you. Now that you have a clearer understanding of what you're dealing with, you can take it step by step, day by day.

You probably have noted what a vital role exercise has in determining your well-being. Starting an aerobic exercise program is very difficult, but the benefits are well worth it. It has done wonders for many people with MVPS/D. Exercise lessens fatigue, lowers resting pulse rates, and decreases chest pains, just to name a few of the benefits it brings in its wake. The same is true of limiting sugar and caffeine intake.

Don't try to change everything all at once, or you certainly will be overwhelmed. Implement the changes you wish to make little by little, and before you know it you will not only begin to see improvements in your symptoms, you will begin to see improvements in your lifestyle.

CHAPTER 4

Psychological Symptoms of Dysautonomia

He who fears he will suffer, already suffers from his fear.

—Montaigne

The word "psychological" often brings up strong feelings in people. Many individuals don't even want to talk about psychological symptoms, especially if they actually have experienced or are experiencing such symptoms. A lot of people think they will be judged as "weaklings" and/or "worthless" if they reveal they suffer from depression or they discuss their chronic anxiety or panic attacks.

Unfortunately, these are nineteenth-century notions that have survived into the twenty-first century. Such ideas ignore all the information we now have about how brain chemistry works. Today, we know quite a lot about the biochemicals that regulate our moods and our emotional lives, and we are learning more every day.

When a particular neurotransmitter is out of whack and causing depression, there is an entire arsenal of antidepressants that can be called upon to restore that individual to an emotionally balanced state. Today, many psychological symptoms are treated just as well as physical symptoms. It is not a sign of weakness to seek help for these symptoms. On the contrary, seeking help is a sign of sanity.

If you have ever thought that your problems are "all in your head," or that you are just not emotionally strong enough to handle life, you are probably wrong. Your symptoms are real and they can be treated effectively. They have nothing to do with being a weak person, either of body or mind.

Psychological Symptoms Associated with MVPS/D

The bulleted list below is a roster of the most common psychological symptoms associated with mitral valve prolapse syndrome/dysautonomia (MVPS/D). Each symptom is discussed in this chapter. The text will address most of the fears that you may be experiencing because of these symptoms. It will provide you with specific helpful information for dealing with your particular set of symptoms, or it will send you to other helpful sources.

- Generalized anxiety disorder (GAD)

- Social phobia

- Specific phobia

- Panic attacks

- Panic disorder

- Depression

Generalized Anxiety Disorder

Martha is a woman who once suffered from Generalized Anxiety Disorder (GAD). The following is her description of her experience with it:

> *I always thought I was just a worrier. I'd feel keyed up and unable to relax. At times, my worries would come and go, and at times they would be with me constantly. I could worry for days on end without being able to relax at all. I'd worry about what I was going to fix for a dinner party, or what would be a great present for somebody. I just couldn't let anything go. I would obsess about something until something else came along to worry about. Then, I would obsess about that.*

Generalized anxiety disorder is the name for feeling much more anxiety than the amount, or degree, of anxiety that most people experience in their daily lives. The person who has GAD feels an *intense* degree of worry and tension *chronically*, even though, to an outside observer, nothing seems sufficiently worrisome to warrant such anxiety.

When you have this disorder, you are always anticipating disaster. You may worry excessively about health, money, family, or work. Sometimes, the true source of your anxiety may be hard to pinpoint. When you have this disorder, the mere thought of getting through an ordinary day may provoke further anxiety.

People with GAD can't seem to shake their worries, even when they realize that their anxiety is more intense than the situation warrants. Also, they seem to be unable to relax. They often have trouble falling asleep or staying asleep. At bedtime, they may feel nauseated, or as though they have a lump in the throat. Many people with GAD also startle more easily than others. Their startle reflex appears to be extremely well developed.

As a rule, however, the impairment associated with GAD is mild. People with the disorder don't feel too restricted in their social settings or on the job. Unlike many other anxiety disorders, those who suffer from GAD, characteristically, don't avoid certain situations as a result of their disorder. However, if severe, GAD can be quite debilitating, making it difficult to carry out even the most ordinary daily activities.

Generalized anxiety disorder comes on gradually and most often strikes people in childhood or adolescence, but it also can begin in the later decades of life. In general, though, the symptoms of GAD seem to diminish with age (National Institute of Mental Health 1999). Successful treatment may include medications such as benzodiazepines (to combat anxiety) or antidepressants. Cognitive-behavioral therapy, relaxation techniques, and biofeedback for controlling muscle tension are also useful.

Social Phobia

Phillip, who suffered from social phobia when he was a young man, described how the disorder affected his life:

> I couldn't go on dates or to parties. For a while I couldn't even go to class. My sophomore year of college, I had to come home for a semester. Before I even left the house, I would be so anxious, and it would escalate as I got closer to class, a party, or whatever. I would feel sick to my stomach. It almost felt as if I had the flu. My heart would pound, my palms would get sweaty, and I would get this feeling of being removed from myself and from everybody else. Whenever I would walk into a room full of people, I'd turn red, and it would feel like everybody's eyes were on me. I was too

embarrassed to stand off in a corner by myself, but I couldn't think of anything to say to anybody. I felt so clumsy. I couldn't wait to get out of wherever I was.

The intense fear of being humiliated in social situations, or, specifically, of embarrassing yourself in front of people is called *social phobia*. This disorder often begins around early adolescence and it seems to run in families (National Institute of Mental Health 1999).

If you suffer from social phobia, when you are in a public place, you tend to think that others are very competent and that you are not. Any small mistakes that you might make will seem much bigger to you than they really are. Furthermore, people with social phobia tend to blush a lot. But if you have social phobia, blushing may seem particularly embarrassing to you, and you may feel as though all eyes are focused on you. You may even be afraid of being with people except for those in your family, or childhood friends.

Your fear may be more specific, e.g., you might feel anxious about giving a speech, talking to your boss (or any other authority figure), or dating. The most common social phobia is the fear of public speaking. Sometimes, social phobia encompasses a generalized fear of social situations, such as going to or being at parties. More rarely it may involve fears of using a public restroom, dining out, talking on the telephone, or writing in the presence of other people, such as when signing a check.

Although this phobia is often thought of as a form of shyness, social phobia and shyness are not the same. Shy people can be very uneasy around others, but they don't experience the extreme anxiety when anticipating a social situation, and they don't necessarily avoid circumstances that make them feel self-conscious. In contrast, people with social phobia aren't necessarily shy at all. Most of the time they can be completely at ease with others, but particular situations, e.g., walking down an aisle in public or making a speech, can cause them to feel intense anxiety.

Social phobia disrupts normal life, interfering with careers or social relationships. For example, someone might turn down a job promotion because he or she is too terrified to give public presentations. The dread of a social event can begin weeks in advance, and its symptoms can be quite debilitating.

People with social phobia are aware that their feelings are irrational. Still, they experience a great deal of dread before facing a feared situation, and they may go out of their way to avoid it. Even if they manage to confront what they fear, they usually feel uncomfortable throughout the confrontation. Afterwards, unpleasant feelings may linger, as they worry about how they might have been judged, or what others might have thought or observed about them.

Many people who suffer from social phobia find relief from their symptoms when treated with cognitive-behavioral therapy or medications, or a combination of the two treatments. Therapy may involve learning to view social events differently by repeated exposure to a seemingly threatening social situation. Eventually, the repetition of exposures to the feared circumstance or event causes the fear to diminish and makes it easier to face the circumstance or event. Therapy may also involve learning anxiety-reducing techniques, new social skills, and relaxation techniques.

Specific Phobias

Here is Martin's account of his specific phobia—the fear of flying:

> *I'm scared to death of flying, and I never do it anymore. It's awful when that airplane door closes, and I feel trapped. My heart pounds, and I sweat bullets. If somebody starts talking to me, I get very stiff and preoccupied. When the airplane starts to ascend, it just reinforces my feeling that I can't get out. I feel trapped. I picture myself losing control, freaking out, climbing the walls; but, of course, I never do. I am not afraid of crashing or hitting turbulence. It's just that feeling of being trapped. Whenever I've thought about changing jobs, I've had to think, "Will I be under pressure to fly?" These days, I only go to places I can get to by driving or taking a train. My friends always point out that I couldn't get off a train traveling at high speeds either, so why don't trains bother me? I just tell them it isn't a rational fear.*

Specific phobias are intense, irrational fears of certain things or situations, such as dogs, closed-in places, heights, escalators, tunnels, being in water, driving on freeways, and flying. Many people experience specific phobias. Those with specific phobias, like Martin, often realize that their fears are irrational. Often, when they must face, or even think about facing, the feared object or situation, it brings on a panic attack or severe anxiety.

If the object of their fear is easy to avoid, people with these phobias may not feel the need to seek treatment. Instead, they will continually avoid the feared object. Sometimes, they make important career or personal decisions based solely on avoiding a phobic situation. This is called *avoidance behavior*.

When phobias interfere with a person's life, treatment can help. Successful treatment usually involves the kind of cognitive-behavioral therapy called *desensitization* or *exposure therapy*, in which patients are gradually exposed to what frightens them until they become accustomed to dealing with their fears, and their fears begin to fade because they no longer have the power to frighten.

Panic Attacks

Jamie had her first panic attack when she was twenty-eight years old. Here's how she described it:

> *I was sitting on the couch watching TV, when suddenly I felt very uncomfortable. My legs were shaking, and I felt scared and anxious for no apparent reason. My heart started to race, and I thought, "I am going to die any second." I wanted to run away from this feeling, but I knew that I couldn't, so I got up and started walking around the house. I was so agitated and uncomfortable that I just kept walking around until this feeling went away about ten minutes later. At the time this was happening, I had no idea I was having a panic attack. I realized that after I talked to a friend of mine who has panic attacks. She made me understand that I was not going crazy.*

For quite some time it has been well documented that there is an association between MVPS/D and panic attacks. The MVP Center in Birmingham, Alabama, found the incidence of panic attacks to be present in 60 percent of their patients who had been diagnosed with MVPS/D (Frederickson 1992).

A great many people will not tell their physicians they have panic attacks, unless they are questioned carefully. Many will deny panic attacks but will admit to "sudden, frightening, smothering spells" that make them think they are dying.

Panic attacks usually occur spontaneously. The symptoms are as follows:

- Shortness of breath

- Rapid heartbeat

- Sweating

- Chest pain

- Intense anxiety accompanied by the urge to flee

- Sometimes feeling out of touch with reality

Attacks occur at various times and places, but most commonly while shopping in a grocery store or driving on the freeway. A nocturnal panic attack can occur during sleep, causing the person to awaken with a feeling of being smothered.

Panic attacks are extremely frightening, and some people immediately adopt new behaviors in their efforts to lessen the likelihood of having another attack. Such behaviors may include avoiding grocery stores, not driving, or developing a fear of sleep and, thus, insomnia. When this avoidance behavior becomes severe, it is known as *agoraphobia*, a condition where the person may be psychologically unable to leave his or her home.

Today, it is well accepted that panic attacks are triggered by certain biochemical imbalances in the central nervous system. People can be treated with medication, which tends to stabilize these biochemical imbalances. If you have suffered panic attacks, your avoidance behaviors may be well established. If that is the case, it is sometimes very helpful to seek the services of a good clinical psychologist or psychiatrist in addition to your medical doctor, to learn how to control the behavioral consequences of the chemical imbalance.

Panic attacks are not life-threatening, but they can be devastating to your lifestyle as well as to your self-confidence. Your family may have a difficult time understanding your behavior, and prolonged problems may be very stressful on your relationships, both at home and at your job (see chapter 9).

Panic Disorder

Panic disorder is probably the most frequently reported psychiatric syndrome associated with MVPS/D (Hamilton 1991). It is manifested by discrete periods of intense fear or discomfort with associated physical and emotional symptoms. The actual panic attacks tend to be fairly short in duration, typically lasting no more than a few minutes. In most instances, these attacks seem to be unrelated to any specific stressor. They seem to come "out of the blue."

Panic attacks are the hallmark of panic disorder. Some people who have one panic attack or an occasional attack in a lifetime never develop a problem serious enough to affect their lives. For others, the attacks continue and develop into full-fledged panic disorder.

As the disorder progresses over time, people who have suffered an attack in specific situations tend to develop an anticipatory fear of those situations. After developing this kind of anticipatory anxiety about a situation, they are then at risk for experiencing a recurrence of attacks in that situation. As a result, they tend to avoid the situations in which they became panic-stricken, and their world becomes more and more enclosed. When people have experienced panic in so many social settings that they become basically housebound, they are then experiencing agoraphobia.

The onset of panic disorder, typically, is during the person's late twenties. Panic disorder with associated agoraphobia is approximately twice as common in women as in men (Hamilton 1991).

Initially, the attacks may be limited in the number of symptoms experienced or in the frequency of the attacks. However, the tendency is for this disorder to progress. This is, in part, because there is a great deal of anticipatory anxiety in the intervals between the attacks. The anticipatory anxiety tends to feed on itself, and as people become more fearful of having an attack, they also become more at risk to have one.

There is a fairly wide variation in the number of symptoms someone may experience during an attack. Some people may experience all of the symptoms listed below, while others may experience only one or two.

Commonly Reported Symptoms of Panic Attacks

- Shortness of breath or feelings of smothering

- Dizziness or faintness

- Palpitations or "racing heart"

- Trembling or shaking

- Sweating

- Choking

- Nausea or abdominal distress

- Numbness or tingling

- Flushing or chills

- Chest pain or discomfort

- Fear of dying

- Fear of going crazy or of losing control

Although experiencing any one of these symptoms can be quite distressing, the presence of four or more of these symptoms is necessary for a diagnosis of panic disorder. Fewer than four symptoms is described as "limited symptom attacks."

People with MVPS/D seem to be at higher risk to develop panic disorder than the general population (Hamilton 1991); however, not all people with MVPS/D will develop the disorder. When someone does develop it, a referral to a psychiatrist is usually in order.

It is extremely important to understand that this referral does not mean that the person's problems are "all in their head." Panic disorder is a very real illness. It is neither imaginary nor self-induced. It is the result of biochemical imbalances and abnormalities in the person's body, and, as such, medications are frequently necessary to treat it properly. Although it can be extremely debilitating, particularly if it progresses and becomes severe, it is quite treatable, and it can be interrupted and controlled in its early stages with effective treatment.

Depression

Carrie went through an episode of depression in 1990. Here is her description of what it was like:

> *I had a wonderful family, a beautiful house, and a husband who loved me, but something didn't feel quite right inside of me. I couldn't figure out what was wrong. Everything I had always loved no longer seemed important to me. I started dreading mornings. As soon as I opened my eyes, this horrible feeling of sadness came over me. I had to force myself to get out of bed and walk to the kitchen. Trying to eat breakfast was even harder. I got to the point where I couldn't finish even one piece of toast. I quickly lost fifteen pounds. Everyday tasks like brushing my teeth or combing my hair were so overwhelming that I just decided to stay in bed for three months. I wouldn't wish this feeling on my worst enemy.*

Depression should not be confused with the occasional feelings of unhappiness that everyone experiences. Those periods of sadness are usually associated with unhappy events like a death in the family, or personal failures, like being turned down for a promotion; or the emotional letdowns that take place around holidays. Grief and sadness are normal and temporary reactions to life's stresses. Time heals these intense feelings, the moods lift, and people continue being able to function.

In contrast, people with depression do not feel better for months, and if they do not receive medical help, sometimes for years. Depression affects feelings, thoughts, behaviors, and physiological functioning. There is a loss of interest in all of the usual activities that provide pleasure, such as sex, work, friends, hobbies, entertainment, and even food.

Symptoms of Depression

- Persistent low, anxious, or "empty" feelings

- Loss of interest or ability to feel pleasure in usual activities, including sex

- Appetite and significant weight changes, either loss or gain

- Feelings of hopelessness and pessimism

- Feelings of guilt, worthlessness, and helplessness

- Recurrent thoughts of death or suicide

- Sleep disturbances (insomnia, early-morning waking, or oversleeping)

- Complaints or evidence of diminished ability to think or to concentrate

In some people, symptoms of depression may begin suddenly and seem to have no apparent relation to what is happening in their lives. Other people appear to have been depressed all their lives. Some people experience only a single episode of depression in their lifetimes, but it is more commonly a recurrent disorder.

Depression is among the most prevalent of the mental disorders, affecting people of all ages, socioeconomic classes, races, and cultures. Fortunately, it is also one of the most responsive to treatment. Almost 80 percent of all serious depressions can be successfully alleviated (Sargent 1994). The choice of treatment for depression typically depends on the pattern, severity, and persistence of symptoms, and the history of the illness.

Some people experience brief depressive episodes with relatively mild symptoms lasting over days. These episodes may cause personal distress and discomfort, but do not seriously interfere with the person's ability to function at work or at home. Often, such episodes improve without intensive treatment, but will be helped by counseling, therapy, and, sometimes, anti-anxiety medication.

If the symptoms of depression listed above continue for weeks and include some interference with work and family activities (the person can carry out usual responsibilities, but with difficulty), a comprehensive diagnostic assessment, including a thorough medical examination, is essential. Medical evaluation is necessary because a variety of physical illnesses can produce or precipitate depression. Once this factor is ruled out, the patient will have a choice of antidepressants and/or therapy. Often, a combination of medication and therapy is the most effective treatment.

More intensive treatment is called for when depression involves thoughts of death, suicide attempts, impaired judgment, and marked mood swings or bipolar (manic depression) tendencies. For these types of depression, antidepressants are usually mandatory.

Treatments are sometimes modified and adjusted to suit the individual need of the patient. Close monitoring is essential to track the patient's response to prescribed medications and to his or her progress.

Seasonal Affective Disorder

Seasonal Affective Disorder (SAD) is a very common problem for people with MVPS/D. This is particularly noticeable in the months from November through March, when many people experience a mild depression known as seasonal affective disorder, or SAD. This disorder is very common in Scandinavian countries in the winter, when there is very little sunlight available during very short days. It is quite puzzling why SAD is so prevalent in people with MVPS/D (Watkins 1990).

Exposure to bright light, known as phototherapy, has been found to be an effective method for treating SAD (Rosenthal 1993). The person with SAD sits in front of a light box for a given time each day. The light box is a specially bright lamp that casts a light which approximates sunlight. Sometimes this treatment is coupled with other methods of treatment similar to those for other depressive disorders. These special light boxes can be purchased from several different companies (see Resources). Note that if your doctor prescribes light therapy, your insurance may pay for it.

Treatment Options for Psychological Symptoms

Treatment should be selected according to the individual needs and preferences of the patient. Any treatment that fails to produce an effect within several months should be reassessed.

- Cognitive-behavioral therapy

- Systematic desensitization (exposure therapy)

- Breathing and relaxation exercises

- Medication

Cognitive-Behavioral Therapy

Cognitive-behavioral therapy combines cognitive therapy, which can teach you to modify or eliminate the thought patterns contributing to your symptoms, and behavioral therapy, which aims at helping you to change your behavior.

Cognitive-behavioral therapy is particularly valuable if you have panic attacks, because it can teach you to anticipate and prepare yourself for those situations and bodily sensations that may trigger your panic attacks. In this type of therapy, the focus is seldom on your past, as is the case with some other forms of psychotherapy. Instead, the dialogue between you and the therapist centers on the difficulties and successes you are experiencing at the present time, and on the skills you need to learn to overcome your present-day problems.

Typically, if you are undergoing cognitive-behavioral therapy, you meet with a therapist for one to three hours a week. During the cognitive part of the therapy, the therapist usually conducts a careful search for the thoughts and feelings that accompany your panic attack symptoms.

The therapist helps you to identify the thinking patterns that lead to your misinterpretation of your own bodily sensations and to your assumption that "the worst" is happening to you. Such patterns of thinking may be deeply ingrained, and it may take a lot of practice; first to "see" the patterns, and then to change them.

The behavioral part of this therapy may involve some systematic training in relaxation techniques. By learning to relax, you may acquire the ability to reduce your generalized anxiety and stress. In addition, the behavioral part of this therapy may include training in systematic desensitization.

Systematic Desensitization (Exposure Therapy)

Systematic desensitization is a gradual form of exposure to real-life situations that frighten you. In this procedure, you progress very slowly, beginning with exposure to an object or situation that is only a little bit frightening, and, gradually, you confront situations that are more fearful.

For example, if you are afraid of water, systematic desensitization would first have you wade in the shallow end of a swimming pool. Then, you would learn to swim some basic strokes while still in the shallow part of the pool. Eventually, you wind up swimming (or floating) in the deep end of the pool, feeling perfectly comfortable. Clearly, this is a process that takes a certain amount of time. But it is a proven therapy for certain types of fear.

If you do not have access to the real object of your fears, such as if you are afraid of thunderstorms, then the therapist may substitute films, or audiovisual tapes of the object or situation that is so frightening. Photographs and models also may be used in this kind of therapy (Greist, Jefferson, and Marks 1986).

Breathing Exercises

A therapist can teach you to do breathing exercises that will calm you and counteract the overbreathing, or hyperventilation, that often occurs during a panic attack. Some people are able to learn one or more of these techniques from someone else who has learned them, or through the use of books.

When most people feel panic, they tend to gasp, take in a breath, and hold onto it. This results in a sensation of fullness and an inability to take in enough air. This, in turn, produces shallow breathing or hyperventilation. The hyperventilation can trigger a panic attack.

Breath training can counteract this entire process. Here is one breathing exercise that individuals with panic disorder or agoraphobia have found to be particularly helpful (adapted from Davis, Eshelman, and McKay 2000).

1. First exhale. Whenever you feel the first sign of nervousness or panic, always exhale. It is essential to exhale first so that

your lungs open up and you will feel as though there is plenty of room to take a good, deep breath.

2. Next, inhale and exhale through your nose. Exhaling through your nose slows down your breathing and prevents hyperventilation. If you cannot exhale through your nose, inhale through your mouth and exhale through your mouth by pretending that you are blowing out through a straw.

3. Then, lie on your back and place one hand over your abdomen and the other hand on your chest. Exhale first, and then breathe in through your nose, counting, "One . . . two . . . three." Pause a second, and then breathe out through your mouth, counting "One . . . two . . . three . . . four." Make sure that your exhalation is always longer than your inhalation. This will keep you from taking short, gasping panic breaths.

4. After you feel comfortable doing step 3, you can slow your breathing even further. Breathe in and count, "One . . . two . . . three . . . four . . . five." Keep practicing these slow, deep breaths, which will push the hand on your abdomen up, but will allow very little movement for the hand on your chest. When your mind drifts, refocus on your breathing.

There are many books that can teach you how to do breathing exercises that will calm you down. *The Relaxation & Stress Reduction Workbook* by Davis, Eshelman, and McKay (2000), from which the exercise above has been adapted, is particularly good, but there are many others available, as well. You also will find more breathing exercises in chapter 11 if you wish to see some now.

Medications

Prescription medications are commonly used for anxiety, panic disorder, and depression. As the medication begins to take effect and people observe that their symptoms are less severe and occur less often, they are increasingly able to venture into situations that were off limits to them. There are several groups of medications to choose from for these purposes.

Beta-Blockers

One such group is called *beta-blockers*. There are many different kinds of beta-blockers available for your physician to select from, and the choice will depend not only on your symptoms, but also on any other contributing medical conditions you might have. Beta-blockers are normally prescribed for treating high blood pressure. Certain beta-blockers also seem to work well for the treatment of social phobia because of their ability to reduce palpitations, sweating, blushing, and trembling. This is due to their ability to cross the blood-brain barrier.

It has been my observation that people with MVPS/D usually require a very small dose of a beta-blocker for it to work well. Note that beta-blockers *cannot* be used by people with severe allergies or asthma. Also, they should be used with caution on people with MVPS/D who demonstrate a slow pulse rate, as their pulse rate would be worsened by a beta-blocker.

Anti-Anxiety Medications

Another group of medicines widely used to combat anxiety disorders is called *anti-anxiety medication*. These medications help to calm and relax the anxious person and to neutralize the troubling symptoms. There are a number of anti-anxiety medications currently available. The preferred types of medication for most anxiety disorders are the benzodiazepines. You may recognize some brand-names of these medications, Klonopin®, Ativan®, and Xanax®, to name but three, are among the most widely used anti-anxiety medications.

In addition to these, an atypical anti-anxiety medication, BuSpar, has been used with some success for generalized anxiety disorders. Benzodiazepines are relatively fast-acting medications. In contrast, BuSpar must be taken daily for two to three weeks before results become noticeable. However, BuSpar offers the benefits of reduced anxiety, without the problems of sedation and potential drug dependence sometimes seen with the benzodiazepines.

As stated, most benzodiazepines will begin to take effect within hours, some in even less time. The dosage will vary a great deal depending on the symptoms and the person's body chemistry.

"In recent years, concern has arisen regarding potential benzodiazepine abuse and dependence. Certainly, people who chronically use benzodiazepines do develop a physiological dependence on these medications. Nonetheless, concerns in both the media and the medical profession may have been overstated. The vast majority of chronically anxious patients do not abuse or become addicted to these medications and rarely require progressive increases in doses. The individuals who do, in fact, present a significant risk of abuse are those with a family history of alcohol or other substance abuses. Benzodiazepines are not appropriate for such people" (Preston, O'Neal, and Talaga 1999).

Antidepressants

Antidepressants are another widely used group of medications. They are used mostly to treat clinical depressions but also can be helpful for mild depressions. Antidepressants, although not "uppers" or stimulants, eliminate or reduce the symptoms of depression and help the depressed person to feel the way she or he used to feel before becoming depressed.

Antidepressants are also used for disorders characterized principally by anxiety. They can block the symptoms of panic, including rapid heartbeat, dizziness, chest pains, nausea, and breathing problems. Antidepressants are also used to treat some phobias.

The physician chooses the particular type of antidepressant to prescribe based on the individual patient's symptoms. As a rule, when someone begins taking an antidepressant, improvement does not begin to show immediately. With most of these medications it takes one to three weeks before changes begin to occur.

These treatments for the psychological aspects of MVPS/D have been touched upon only briefly. For proper treatment for the psychological aspects of your own MVPS/D, you must see a physician to diagnose and prescribe what will be the most suitable option for you. Proper treatment is the key to getting your life back under control.

All of the different types of medications will be more thoroughly discussed in chapter 10. Many people hate even the thought of taking medication, either because they are afraid of side effects, or because they feel they are somehow "weaker" if they have to rely on a drug to make them feel better. The same is true of going to a therapist. In our society there is still a terrible stigma attached to seeing a psychiatrist. This issue, too, will be addressed in chapter 10.

Unfortunately, there is no magic pill that, upon ingestion, will cause all of the symptoms of MVPS/D you may be experiencing to disappear. But proper treatment may also require lifestyle changes on your part. Therefore, lifestyle modifications, dietary changes, and behavior modification techniques may all be in order to maximize the treatment your doctor prescribes for you. Chapters 5 through 11 will discuss these issues in detail and at some length. Education, exercise, and a sense of humor also will be stressed. In the next chapters, you will read about success stories and how they were accomplished. Although, at the moment, it may seem impossible to deal with because of its complexity, you will learn that it is indeed possible to cope with MVPS/D.

CHAPTER 5

The Many Ways in Which Dysautonomia Affects Your Life

Man is not disturbed by events, but by the view he takes of them.

—Epictetus

"While mitral valve prolapse syndrome/dysautonomia (MVPS/D) is not life-threatening, it may be lifestyle-threatening," says Lyn Frederickson, author of *Confronting Mitral Valve Prolapse Syndrome.* Truer words could not be spoken. Mitral valve prolapse syndrome/dysautonomia (MVPS/D) can definitely have an impact on your lifestyle. Until you get your autonomic nervous system back in balance, having MVPS/D can alter the way you feel, the way you think, the way you act, and the way you go about your daily life.

Self-Esteem and Self-Confidence

How you view yourself defines your self-esteem and your self-confidence. Unfortunately, low self-esteem and low self-confidence are often characteristics of those with MVPS/D (Rippetoe 1993).

If you are hard on yourself when you make a mistake, if you don't like what you see in the mirror, or if you think you are a failure every time you feel anxious, the chances are good that you have low self-esteem. If you have low self-esteem, you probably don't like yourself all that much, and if you don't like yourself, the following statement may be hard to believe: Believe it or not, *coping with*

MVPS/D is possible. To find out whether you have low self-esteem ask yourself these questions:

- Do you often feel unsure of yourself?

- Do others seem to enjoy life more than you do?

- Do you often think that people think negatively of you?

- Do you feel self-conscious when you are in public places?

- Do you put yourself down?

- Do you feel misunderstood?

- Do you usually keep quiet in groups even when you have something to say?

If you answered "yes" to some of these questions, you may have a problem with self-confidence. For example, here is how Jennifer feels about the issue of her self-esteem and the fact that she has MVPS/D:

> *I've had symptoms of MVPS/D since I was five years old. I always felt different from the other kids at school. They looked like they were having so much fun, while I could hardly wait to get home. This anxious feeling stayed with me every day, all the way through high school. I had so much anxiety at school. I worried about teachers calling on me and kids laughing at me if I gave the wrong answer. I know these anxieties contributed to my low self-esteem.*
>
> *In those days I didn't know anything about MVPS/D. I just thought I must be "weaker" than everyone else. It was only after growing up and finding out about MVPS/D and realizing that I was not a weak, inferior person that I was able to build up my self-esteem and self-confidence.*

Anxiety and low self-esteem can create a vicious cycle. Perhaps years of battling your MVPS/D have led to you having low self-esteem. It doesn't really matter which came first because either way, the two are feeding on each other now. Alleviating one problem won't necessarily help the other, but working on both will bring you further along the road to coping with your MVPS/D.

Be Kind to Yourself

Low self-esteem doesn't change to high self-esteem overnight. Nevertheless, being good to yourself and feeling compassion for yourself will start helping immensely. You can practice being kind to yourself every day by becoming more conscious of how you "speak" to yourself. If you have low self-esteem, there's a good chance that your self-talk is full of phrases like, "You are such a fool." "You always mess up." "No wonder, you are worried about _____ [fill in the blank]. You are so stupid, that you are bound to fail." And so on. If you talk to yourself in this fashion, the odds are good that you are much harder on yourself than you are on other people.

Would you get angry with someone else for being anxious? Of course not. Then why be angry with yourself? Think of the words you use to comfort your friends when they are troubled by fear and anxiety, and minister to yourself the same way. This is a technique you can try whenever you're having critical thoughts about yourself. Try to talk to yourself the way you would to a friend. At first, you may not believe those comforting words, but time and practice will make a difference.

The main difficulty with changing low self-esteem is recognizing the problem in the first place. You may not even notice when you're being hypercritical of yourself. You might not see the connection between your self-criticism and your constant anxiety. Take the time to observe how you talk to yourself. What you say to yourself when you talk to yourself can be very informative about your state of mind.

Keeping a Journal

One way to become more aware of the kind of self-talk you engage in is to write down some of your thoughts in a notebook or journal. Whenever you find yourself thinking about your problems, try to record what goes on in your mind by writing down your thoughts. Forget grammar, spelling, and punctuation. Just try to follow the words in your head and get them down on paper. Try this for a week (or a month).

When you have made a few entries recording your negative self-talk, then, using the same notebook, write down all the kind, comforting words you can say to yourself instead of beating yourself up. Use the same kind of nurturing, caring language that you would with a good friend.

For example, suppose you wrote about an event where you just "knew" that you had made a fool of yourself. You could plan to add some nurturing language to your original entry immediately. That way, you would be at least as kind to yourself as you would to a friend.

Your journal entry might go something like this: "I should never have tried to speak at the P.T.A. meeting in favor of passing the new school bond. I made a perfect fool of myself. I was so anxious, I started out mumbling, and my voice was so low, no one could hear me. The chairwoman had to ask me to raise my voice at least four times. Then, when I finally got loud enough, my voice cracked because I care so much about the issue. It was so embarrassing. I feel as if I had humiliated myself in front of the whole P.T.A."

After writing an entry like that, you could add something like this: "Well, at least I got my point across. By the time I sat down, everyone had heard what I had to say. My presentation may have left a lot to be desired, but when I was through speaking, I had brought some important new information to the discussion. I am not a professional public speaker, but I got some very complex information out to the people who needed to hear it. No one else even tried to do what I did. And, no matter how hard it was for me to do, I think I succeeded."

Strategies to Develop Confidence

- **Emphasize your strengths.** Give yourself credit for everything you try. Many people with MVPS/D are very quick to criticize themselves when they try something new and they don't succeed immediately. They focus on their limitations. You must learn to be just as quick to focus on your strengths, and to give yourself credit for the fact that you tried something new. By focusing on what you can do, you praise yourself for your efforts, rather than emphasizing only the results. Starting from the base of what you can do instead of what you *should* do helps you to live within the bounds of your inevitable limitations.

- **Take risks.** People with MVPS/D often seem to have an extremely difficult time accepting change and new challenges in their life. Approach new experiences as opportunities to learn rather than occasions to win or lose. Doing this opens you up to new possibilities and can increase your sense of self-acceptance. Not doing this turns every possibility into an opportunity for failure, and thus inhibits your personal growth.

- **Use self-talk.** For example, when you catch yourself expecting perfection, remind yourself that you can't do everything perfectly, that it's only possible to try to do things and to try to do them well. This allows you to accept yourself while still striving to improve.

Guilt

Guilt is the inability to forgive yourself for a perceived wrong-doing. A *perceived wrongdoing* means that you *believe* you have done something wrong. The perceived wrong may have been an action, a thought, or a feeling. If it was an action, you probably think of it as a mistake. You feel guilty for doing the wrong because you cannot forgive yourself. You cannot let it go. If you cannot forgive yourself, you will not overcome the guilt.

You may feel guilty about not being able to do certain things because of your MVPS/D symptoms. For example, if you cannot attend an important social function, such as going to the opening of a play that your child is performing in at school, because of your anxiety, or you cannot take your kids somewhere because of your fear of driving, you may feel terribly guilty afterwards.

Your children, especially, may know how to press your buttons and make you feel guilty. Your family and friends may cause you to feel even more guilty because of their lack of knowledge about MVPS/D. To make matters worse, you may start to make up elaborate stories when you can't accomplish certain tasks, and then you feel guilty about making up those stories. Finally, you may find yourself feeling guilty about having MVPS/D.

Accepting that you have MVPS/D is essential for moving on to control it. Also, you may need to accept your MVPS/D in order to be strong in the face of the negativity you receive from family and friends. If you don't accept that you have it, you will not be able to discuss it with them. A frank and full discussion of your needs and limitations with all those who care about you can go a long way toward creating the kind of support you need, and it also can go a long way toward alleviating your feelings of guilt.

Assertiveness

Do you often find that other people have coerced you into thinking their way? Is it difficult for you to express your positive or negative feelings openly and honestly? Do you sometimes lose control and become angry at people who have not done anything to warrant your anger?

Answering "yes" to any of these questions may be your expression of a common problem known as "lack of assertiveness." Being assertive involves asking for what you want (or saying "no") in a simple, direct fashion that does not negate, attack, or manipulate anyone else. When you are *aggressive*, you do negate, attack, and try to manipulate others. But when you are *assertive*, you communicate what you want honestly and forthrightly. When you are assertive, others do not feel uncomfortable with you because you are not hiding anything from them. You receive respect in exchange for your honesty.

Assertiveness does not make demands or give orders. It makes plain and simple statements and requests, such as this to your supervisor, "I believe I have earned a promotion," or this to a waiter, "I think the addition on my bill is not correct. Would you mind doing it once more?" Becoming more assertive can be particularly helpful when dealing with physicians, family, and friends who don't know anything about MVPS/D, and don't understand the complexity of your symptoms.

As a rule, people with MVPS/D care a great deal about making other people happy, sometimes at their own expense. More than likely they also have a little more trouble than most people in expressing their negative emotions, for fear of hurting or offending others.

In the words of clinical psychologist E. J. Bourne:

Developing assertiveness begins with an awareness of your own needs—knowing what it is you want. Then you need to learn that it's okay to meet your needs without feeling selfish or fearing disapproval. You become assertive, finally, when *you know you have the right to ask for what you want.* You are conscious of your basic rights as a human being and *you are willing to exercise those rights* (Bourne 2001, p. 74, emphasis in original).

Strategies for Developing Self-Assertiveness

- **Be as specific and as clear as possible about what you want, think, and feel.** The following types of statements project this precision: "I want to. . . ," "I don't want you to. . . ," "I have a different opinion. I think that. . . ." It can be helpful to explain exactly what you mean and exactly what you don't mean. This is especially true when dealing with your doctors, because they are not mind readers, and they need to know what it is that you want, think, and feel.

- **Be direct**. Deliver your message to the person for whom it is intended. If you want to tell Jane something, tell Jane. Do not tell everyone except Jane, and do not tell a member of a group that Jane also attends.

- **"Own" your message**. Acknowledge that your message comes from your frame of reference, your concepts of good versus bad and right versus wrong, and your perceptions. You can acknowledge ownership with personalized "I" statements such as, "I don't agree with you," as opposed to "You're wrong," or "I'd like you to mow the lawn," as opposed to "You really should mow the lawn, you know." Suggesting that someone is wrong or bad, and should change for her/his own benefit will only foster resentment and resistance rather than understanding and cooperation.

As you learn to be more assertive, remember to use your assertiveness techniques selectively. It is not only what you say to someone verbally, it is also how you communicate nonverbally with your voice tones, hand gestures, eye contact, facial expression, and body posture that influences how others perceive you.

Fears and Phobias

Phobias are persistent, irrational fears of certain objects or situations. They manifest in different forms. The fear associated with a phobia can focus on a particular object (specific phobia) or be a fear of embarrassment in a public setting (social phobia). People with MVPS/D often suffer from two or more phobias at the same time.

Drawing the distinction between a reasonable fear and the singular terror of a phobia is not always easy. For example, flying into a storm or easing into weaving traffic on a freeway is a reasonable fear. However, a true phobia presents a whole different order of terror. A true phobia is like a wildfire in your central nervous system that's impossible to mistake.

Jan was diagnosed with MVP approximately twenty years ago. Her story is a good example of the difference between a reasonable fear and a phobia. It illustrates the lengths that someone with a real phobia will go through to avoid facing the feared object or situation.

When Jan was in the hospital in labor with her first child, her doctor determined that she needed to have a test done. The testing equipment was on the fifth floor and Jan had a room on the second floor. Taking the test posed a problem for Jan because she was terrified of taking elevators. The nurses tried to convince her that one of them would always be at her side, and all that Jan needed to do was to sit in a wheelchair for the duration of the quick ride up three floors. She refused to hear of it.

Instead, Jan waited until everyone had left her room. Then, between contractions, she proceeded to walk/crawl to the stairs and somehow, on her hands and knees, she managed to make it up the three flights to take the test. After the test, she got back down to her room the same way. This incident convinced Jan to enroll in a course of exposure therapy to conquer her fear of elevators (see chapter 4).

When you suffer from a phobia, you may often experience the fear of imminent death, accompanied by an overwhelming need to flee from whatever has triggered your fear. Furthermore, you may spend a lot of your time dreading your next encounter with the object of your fear, and developing elaborate strategies intended to avoid it.

Avoidance Behavior

More than likely avoidance behavior is the strategy you rely on to ease your discomfort. Unfortunately, the harder you work to avoid the things you fear, the more your brain becomes convinced that the threat is real. This avoidance behavior, similar to that in those who have panic disorder, eventually can develop into full-blown agoraphobia, which is the inability to go beyond known and safe surroundings because of intense anxiety. The "rituals" you may perform to reduce your anxiety may just make matters worse.

Donna's story provides a typical example of avoidance behavior.

Donna dreaded public speaking. Unfortunately for her, giving an oral speech was a requirement of several classes she was taking in school. Donna did everything she could to get out of giving these speeches. Twice, she lied about having laryngitis. She even dropped a few classes rather than speak publicly. Once, when Donna was scheduled to give a speech, she didn't go to school for three weeks. Then she went to her instructor's office and told him that she had missed his class because she had had an emergency appendectomy. She finally graduated without ever giving a speech. Years later, after going through behavioral therapy, Donna is able to speak to groups of people about her experiences with phobias and MVPS/D.

Some people with phobias, particularly social phobias, also may have problems with substance abuse. Like all other anxiety disorders, phobias can cause a double whammy of psychic pain: first from the experience of the condition, and then from the shame of having the condition.

One psychological treatment for people with MVPS/D is to desensitize their phobic response. Social phobia can be effectively treated with medications including antidepressants and anti-anxiety drugs. People with a specific form of social phobia called "performance phobia" are helped by a class of drugs called beta-blockers.

There is no proven drug treatment for specific phobias, but certain medications may help reduce symptoms of anxiety before you have to face a phobic situation. Exposure therapy (see chapter 4) is also a very useful treatment for phobias. It involves helping you to become gradually more comfortable with situations that frighten you. Relaxation and breathing techniques are also helpful (see chapter 2).

Driving

For reasons that are still unknown, the fear of driving is a fairly common phobia among people with MVPS/D. It has been found that exposure therapy is one of the best ways to overcome this phobia. Cruising in a convertible across the Golden Gate Bridge is a scene made famous in many movies, and for many visitors it embodies California's "autocentric" lifestyle. But for people with a driving phobia, merging onto a freeway filled with fast-moving traffic can induce an anxiety attack, and confronting a bridge can be their worst nightmare come true.

It is believed that people with driving phobias subconsciously "overprepare" for emergency physical activity (Weidenbach 2000). Their bodies react to their perceived stress by inhaling more oxygen and exhaling more carbon dioxide than they currently need, which is defined as *hyperventilation*. For some people, the sensations resulting from hyperventilation make them feel even more anxious.

This is Mike's account of his experience with his fear of driving and exposure therapy:

I honestly didn't believe that anything could help me conquer my fear of driving, but I thought I'd give exposure therapy a try. I felt ridiculous at first, because, at your first session, you just sit in the driver's seat as a way of getting used to being in that position. Once you're totally comfortable doing that, then you can move on to the next step, which is starting the car. Only when you're totally comfortable with starting the car, can you actually start driving, but you can only drive very short distances at one time. You never move on to the next step until the previous step feels like second nature to you. I know this sounds too simple, but I am living proof that it works. Believe me, if someone like me can conquer this phobia, I truly feel that anyone can, whether or not they have MVPS/D.

Fear of Medication

Many physicians have reported about their struggles with patients who will not take prescribed medication either orally, or by injection. When they refuse to take their prescribed medications, most of these patients are labeled as "noncompliant," "doctor shoppers," "hostile-dependent," or even as having "passive-aggressive personalities." Most of these patients, however, are not "noncompliant," "doctor shoppers," "hostile-dependent," "passive-aggressive" or any other pejorative name. They simply are afraid to take medication, or, to put it another way, they are medication-phobic.

Medication phobia is a specific phobia where the fear is the delivery of an unknown substance, the medication, to your body, to which you anticipate an adverse reaction. Or the fear may be about a known medication that produces side effects that you have already labeled as dangerous.

Research (Rippetoe 1997) has indicated that if you have medication phobia, you are less likely to seek medical, dental, and/or surgical care, and when you do, you are less likely to comply with treatment and more likely to experience the symptoms of your condition longer than the average patient. This, in turn, creates further fear and a sense of hopelessness about being able to cope with your MVPS/D symptoms.

A lot of people with MVPS/D, who are already prone to anxiety, are sensitized to adverse sensations in their bodies. They are extremely vigilant about how their bodies function, about the subtle sensations their bodies feel, and to signs that their bodies might be betraying them. Feeling a sense of equilibrium makes everyone feel safe and in control. But people with MVPS/D feel that they must be hypervigilant to retain their sense of equilibrium, and they are wary about ingesting anything that could disturb that hard-won sense.

For example, many of you probably feel compelled to read all the information that's included in the insert with your prescription medication. Some of this information can frighten you so much that you may decide not to take the medication. Although it is wise to be a knowledgeable consumer, you really need to be a medical professional to interpret the information included in these inserts in order to put the information in its proper context. The same is true for those of you who keep *The Physician's Desk Reference* in your home.

You may avoid unfamiliar medications to ensure that nothing beyond your control can lead to a situation that will feel risky, one in which the way your body functions is no longer predictable. ("I don't know what my body is going to do; therefore I am at risk. Something terrible might happen.") With this kind of reasoning, your phobia protects you and makes you feel safe, but at the same time, allowing the phobia to govern your actions may be putting your health at risk by causing you to delay and/or avoid proper treatment.

For people with medication phobia, therapy is the most helpful approach. You undergo a short-term desensitization process, designed to reduce fear and sensitivity to an object or circumstance. The therapy may include exposing you to medication in a controlled setting, such as a doctor's or therapist's office, or in the presence of a trusted relative or friend. The medication is introduced to your body in very small amounts until you feel comfortable with any of the possible sensations produced, and until you are convinced those sensations are harmless.

If you know for sure that the idea of taking certain medications makes you uncomfortable, ask your physician for alternatives. For example, most MVPS/D patients who need anesthesia for a surgical procedure request 3-percent carbacaine as a local anesthesia because it contains no epinephrine (adrenaline).

Most health care professionals are happy to work with you to circumvent your fears, if you will only confide your anxieties about new medications to them. Instead of not taking a medication that has been prescribed for you, discuss your fears about that medication with your doctor. This would be a much more successful strategy that can lead to improved health care for you and an enhanced relationship with your doctor.

Fear of Flying

As everyone probably realizes the fear of flying is one of the most common phobias. It occurs in those with MVPS/D and in those without MVPS/D. Some of the reasons people are afraid to fly are the fear of having a panic attack, the fear of being in closed-in spaces, and the fear of crashing, being out of control, or being trapped.

Even though many people are afraid to fly, a very small percentage of people seek help for this fear. For those who do confront this phobia, the task of learning to be more comfortable while flying often takes significant encouragement and an extra dose of effort. Here are some steps you can take to increase your sense of safety when flying:

Strategies to Reduce the Fear of Flying

1. Start by reducing your caffeine and sugar intake on the day before and the day of your flight.

2. Drink lots of water or fruit juice to avoid dehydration from the dry air in the plane.

3. Refrain from drinking alcohol before or during the flight.

4. When the seatbelt sign goes off, stand and stretch or take a walk.

A person who overcomes the fear of flying still knows that anything could go wrong with the flight, just as someone driving a car surely knows that an accident could happen at any time. Therefore, what this person has overcome is the escalating spiral of symptoms triggered by one or more of the anxiety-provoking components of airplane flight. Even though none of us is ever "in control" of anything, we can learn to be "in command" of our thoughts and feelings, and we can trust in something greater than ourselves—more so than we think we can.

Perfectionism

Perfectionism is another common psychological characteristic of people with MVPS/D (Rippetoe 1993). Perfectionism has been defined as the "tendency to have unrealistically high expectations about yourself, others, and life itself" (Bourne 2001, p. 91). When you are a perfectionist, anything that does not meet your standards disappoints and frustrates you. Perfectionism can lead you to "focus excessively on small flaws or mistakes in yourself or your accomplishments. In emphasizing what's wrong, you tend to discount and ignore what's right" (Bourne 2001, p. 91).

When everything you do doesn't measure up to some impossibly high standard you set for yourself, you will experience chronic stress and become burnt-out. When your tendency toward perfectionism is in high gear, you keep telling yourself that you *should*, or you *must*, or you *have to* do whatever it is that you are doing. You may pay no attention to your true desires; they become irrelevant when compared to your desire to do what you *should* do. Moreover, the more perfectionism you practice in your life, the greater the likelihood will be that you will feel intense frustrations and anxieties.

One of the authors of this book, Cheryl Durante, described how being a perfectionist drove her to the point of exhaustion:

> *About twenty years ago, I took a job transcribing legal depositions at home. This was in the days before personal home computers. I actually had to use a typewriter and carbon paper. I wanted my first deposition to be perfect. I wanted my boss to see how good a typist I was. I was determined that my deposition would have few, if any, "typos" in it. Well, to make a long story short, I ended up using an entire ream of paper, 500 sheets to be exact, to type what turned out to be a fifty-page deposition, just so there wouldn't be any "typos" in it.*
>
> *Sitting in that chair all day typing away, I made many of my MVPS/D symptoms much worse. I had tachycardia from not drinking all day, my back went out from sitting in the same position for hours on end without moving anything except my wrists and fingers, and I was totally exhausted. I learned a valuable lesson from that experience. I now set realistic goals and try not to worry about every single mistake I make when working on a project.*

To overcome perfectionism you must make a basic change in how you approach life in general, and how you think about yourself. The following guidelines will provide a starting point for making such a basic change.

Strategies for Overcoming Perfectionism

- **Do not set unattainable goals for yourself**. Sometimes, it's easy to know when you are day-dreaming or indulging in fantasy. At other times, it's hard to know whether a goal is realistic or is an unattainable day-dream. In some instances, it is helpful to discuss your long-term goals with a good friend or a counselor. Such a person can provide you with a "reality check," and help you to adjust your goals in the light of the talents you have exhibited and the resources that are available to you. Another good way to check how realistic your goals are would be to ask yourself this question: "Could anyone else meet these goals that I am setting for myself?" If the answer is "No," then ask yourself why you should be able to attain the goal. If you can't come up with a good answer, then the goal is probably not a realistic one.

- **Do not exaggerate the importance of small mistakes**. Perfectionists constantly beat themselves up for tiny errors that have few if any consequences. In the vast majority of cases, the small mistakes you make will be forgotten in a very short time. Remember that you cannot learn how to do anything without making some mistakes. The errors we make are like tools—we can use them to teach ourselves how to do the job right.

- **Do get involved with the process**. Try not to worry about the end results of whatever job you are doing. Concentrate on the *process* of doing it. As in sports like tennis, basketball, and softball, or games like Scrabble and chess, if you play for the love of the process, instead of concentrating all of your energies on winning, you will have a much better time. You will also have a better likelihood of winning.

Obsessions with Thoughts of Death

People with MVPS/D are often very fearful. They avoid doing anything that carries even the slightest risk of injury. Furthermore, they are often hypervigilant about their health. They may be afraid that even the smallest symptom is a warning sign of a terminal illness. The fear of flying or driving often relates to fear of injury or death. This issue can also take the form of excessive worry about the welfare of loved ones.

Whenever fear leads you to being overcautious, it severely limits your options and activities. It also drains all of the pleasure from your life, and can leave you feeling an empty bitterness. Being over-cautious leads to seeing the world as a fundamentally dangerous place, and limits your participation in most of life's pleasures. Furthermore, if you do not go out into the world and actively engage in some productive activity, you will most likely encounter the problem of having to deal with extreme boredom.

We all know that we are going to die. Most of us also know that we are likely to experience some pain or injuries along the way. Those who limit their lives because of fear of illness or death need to learn to fully accept the fact of their own mortality. No insurance company sells insurance that protects any of us from calamities, much less from death. Learning to accept these "facts of life" is essential for mental health and well-being. Trying to ignore them only creates a sense of greater vulnerability and leaves you unable to take even the slightest of risks.

Fatigue

Clearly, the most common symptoms of MVPS/D are fatigue and malaise, a general sense of not feeling well. The fatigue means you have less energy and strength to engage in normal activities. Your fatigue seems to worsen with exposure to sun, heat, cold, unusual physical exertion, or emotional turmoil. It usually persists over long intervals of time, and is thus distinguishable from the fatigue associated with an acute illness, such as a cold or flu. See chapter 8 for a more complete discussion of fatigue and the issues it brings in its wake.

Panic Attacks

It's easy for most people to advise someone in a "tizzy" not to panic over something, and probably it's almost as easy for that person to calm down with a bit of time, advice, or some conversation with a friend or relative. But for most people with MVPS/D, the panic they experience is far more disabling and difficult to resolve than the occasional feeling of being overwhelmed by responsibilities or events.

Panic, for those of you with MVPS/D, means the possibility of having a *panic attack*, which is the sudden, inexplicable feeling of terror accompanied by a barrage of distressing physical symptoms, and the fear of dying or of losing your mind. See chapter 9 for a thorough discussion of panic attacks.

Depression

Seventy percent of people with MVPS/D suffer from depression (Watkins 1998). Often, when people get their panic attacks under control, it becomes evident that they are also having depressive symptoms. Remember, depression is more than feeling blue or having the "blahs." It is far more than the normal, everyday ups and downs. When your "down" mood lasts for more than a few weeks, your condition may be clinical depression.

Any change, serious loss, or stress such as a divorce, the death of a loved one, the loss of a job, or a move to a new home, can trigger depressive feelings. In most cases these feelings are temporary, but some people, especially those who have a preexisting vulnerability, may develop a depressive illness. Their low mood and depressive symptoms never abate. If that occurs, they need treatment.

Clinical depression is a serious health problem that affects the total person. In addition to the bad feelings and moods, it changes behavior, physical health and appearance, and the ability to handle everyday decisions and pressures. Clinical depression is an illness that requires treatment because its symptoms affect nearly every aspect of living. Without proper treatment, it can become much worse. It can turn into pervasive despair that colors everything black and grim, and makes living a normal life impossible.

What Causes Depression?

All of the causes of depression are not yet known, but there seem to be both biological and emotional factors that increase the likelihood that a person will develop depression. Central to most hypotheses about the causes of depression is the role of the *neurotransmitters,* those biochemicals that transmit signals between the nerve cells of the brain. By means of this signaling, neurotransmitters set in motion the complex interactions that govern our behaviors, feelings, and thoughts. It is currently thought that clinical depression is related to a chemical imbalance of these neurotransmitters. Antidepressant medication helps to correct this imbalance.

It also seems that depression runs in families. Bad life experiences and certain personality traits such as difficulty handling stress, low self-esteem, or extreme pessimism about the future can increase the chances of becoming depressed.

Treatment for Depression

The diagnosis of depression is essential to both patients and physicians, as this is the necessary first step toward treatment. The symptoms can be relieved with psychological therapies, medications, or a combination of both. However, the most important step toward treating depression, and sometimes the most difficult step to take, is to ask for help.

Psychotherapy

A psychotherapist is a medical professional trained to help you understand any psychological illnesses you may have, and to teach you how to deal with them. Talking with a therapist can provide you with valuable support. Psychotherapists can teach you to modify your thought patterns in order to gain more control over your depression. This can be done through cognitive-behavioral therapy. Cognitive restructuring, that is, changing any distorted thought processes you may have, is generally used in combination with a variety of behavioral techniques. Those techniques include breathing retraining, and other activities that target exposure to your bodily sensations.

Antidepressant Medications

As mentioned above, antidepressants relieve the symptoms of depression by correcting a chemical imbalance in the levels of brain chemicals, such as the neurotransmitters (e.g., serotonin) in the brain's nerve cells. The most commonly prescribed antidepressants are the selective serotonin reuptake inhibitors (SSRIs).

- SSRIs generally have fewer side effects associated with the older classes of antidepressants. In some patients, SSRIs may cause headaches, nausea, agitation, changes in sexual functioning, and insomnia. Some of these effects may diminish with time.

- Tricyclic antidepressants are as effective as the SSRIs but have a higher frequency of side effects, including blurred vision, weight gain, dry mouth, and dizziness.

- MAOIs (monoamine oxidase inhibitors) are prescribed much less frequently than SSRIs or tricyclics because of their side effects. MAOIs cannot be taken with certain drugs and foods.

Healing

Healing is more than just bringing a disease under control. It includes finding new strategies to deal with psychological stumbling blocks, it encompasses thoughtful reflection of your life, and putting your depression in perspective. Healing requires accepting your past and having hope for your future.

One area of promise lies in understanding the genetics of depression. Just in the last decade, remarkable progress has been made with brain imaging. The technological capability for defining the structural and functional abnormalities involved in depression is increasing every year. Eventually, advances in medical technolgy will give doctors a better handle on how to treat depression.

The future is bright and the possibilities are many for applying these new capabilities in psychiatry. When scientists can say, "This is the gene (or genes) that causes depression," that will have a tremendous impact on the public. Then, people will really believe that depression is a biologically determined illness. That will have a great beneficial effect on the stigma of behavioral problems and psychiatric disorders.

Gynecological Issues

Many women with MVPS/D are concerned about gynecological problems and whether or not their MVPS/D symptoms will have an impact on these problems. The most frequently asked questions about women's issues are discussed below.

Premenstrual Syndrome

Premenstrual syndrome (PMS) is characterized by symptoms that occur in a cyclical pattern present for anywhere from a few days to two weeks before menstruation. The symptoms usually subside with the onset of menstruation.

The symptoms of PMS include mood swings, feelings of fatigue and/or depression, headaches, backaches, irritability, and forgetfulness. You may also gain weight, feel bloated, and crave sweet and/or salty foods. As you can see, the symptoms of PMS overlap the symptoms of MVPS/D. Therefore, women with MVPS/D can especially benefit from the prescription for PMS below.

Rx for PMS

- **Exercise**: Exercise in general is good for all women. Aerobic exercise can reduce symptoms associated with PMS.

- **Calcium**: The American Journal of Gynecology (2000) confirms earlier suggestions that this mineral is effective at alleviating both physical and psychological symptoms. Nevertheless, you should consult your physician about this before taking calcium supplements.

- **Dietary modifications**: Consume more vitamin B6 and vitamin E, as well as eliminating caffeine, nicotine, and alcohol from your diet. Of course, people with MVPS/D should always abstain from consuming caffeine, nicotine, and alcohol because these substances exacerbate MVPS/D symptoms, including mood swings. Many women say that during PMS, mood swings are the most difficult symptoms with which to deal. Taking vitamins B6 and E may alleviate this symptom.

- **Selective serotonin reuptake inhibitors (SSRIs)**: Prozac, Zoloft, and Paxil. These drugs have become the first-line drug therapy for PMS. It appears they are all equally effective and may relieve PMS in the next monthly cycle following their usage. These medications may alleviate not only mood swings in MVPS/D and PMS, but also the increased anxiety, depression, and carbohydrate craving that can accompany PMS.

- **Anti-anxiety medications**: Xanax, a benzodiazepine, appears to dampen the brain's response to excitability, which is triggered by PMS. Therefore, Xanax may be effective for diminishing symptoms of PMS. Benzodiazepines may quickly reduce the increased anxiety that accompanies PMS. If you need only this type of medication during PMS, you may be able to take it on an as-needed basis. Consult your doctor.

- **Birth control pills**: These may be prescribed to help PMS symptoms for some women. Consult your physician about the pros and cons of taking birth control pills. Certain types of birth control pills are better than others for MVPS/D and for PMS. You need to discuss your particular symptoms with your physician so that you can weigh the benefits and risks of taking birth control pills.

Menopause

Menopause can be a confusing and frustrating time for women, especially women who also have MVPS/D, as they struggle with "what is causing what." Perimenopause and menopause have physical, emotional, and psychological dimensions. Therefore, for many of you, menopause may be a physiological event that triggers MVPS/D symptoms (Hoffman 1997).

The vast majority of people with MVPS/D have a serotonin imbalance (Hamilton 1997). As a rule, the more serotonin we have in our circulation, the better our mood. It is also known that estrogen affects serotonin. Simply put, low estrogen means loss of serotonin. Because people with MVPS/D already have diminished amounts of serotonin, menopause can definitely exacerbate their symptoms.

So should you take estrogen? Estrogen seems to have an effect similar to that of the antidepressant SSRIs. You also need to consider whether you are at risk for osteoporosis, heart disease, breast cancer, and uterine cancer. Furthermore, you should take into consideration how strongly you are affected by your MVPS/D symptoms. You must understand your own health risks and concerns. Balance the pros and cons of the available therapies, then you and your physician can select the therapy that will work best for your individual body's needs.

Infertility

It is believed that there may be a connection between MVPS/D and infertility problems (Watkins 1995). An extraordinary number of women with MVPS/D also seem to have infertility problems (Watkins 1995). Much more research needs to be done on this topic.

Pregnancy

Many women worry about exacerbating their symptoms if they become pregnant. In fact, such worry is not warranted because most women feel much better during pregnancy because they have increased blood volume (Watkins 1995). This increased volume alleviates many MVPS/D symptoms (Watkins 1995).

Personal Accounts

The following section offers two very personal stories from two people's lifetime struggles with MVPS/D and all of its complexities. These accounts are intended to show you that you are not alone, and, more importantly, that there is life after MVPS/D.

Cheryl's Story

I was diagnosed with MVPS/D in 1988. I was really happy to get a diagnosis, because after years of seeing many different kinds of doctors, I was actually glad when one finally found something wrong with me, but I still didn't quite understand everything that was involved with my diagnosis. Frankly, I was just happy to receive any diagnosis.

A few months after getting that diagnosis, I learned there was a book about MVPS/D. I ordered it immediately, and the day it arrived I read it cover to cover (Frederickson 1992). I can't describe how I felt after reading it. I could not believe what I had just read. It was the story of my life.

There was one page in the book that listed most of the major and minor symptoms of the syndrome. I believe there were thirty-two. I had all but one of them. I don't have fainting spells. So, obviously, I had a lot of work to do to get my nervous system back into balance.

The first thing I needed to do was to stop the panic attacks I had recently begun having. I was so frightened by them, and so worried I was either going crazy or going to die, that I couldn't concentrate yet on exercising, increasing my fluid intake, or any of the other beneficial treatments for the syndrome.

I was a nervous wreck. I felt agitated twenty-four hours a day. I couldn't do anything alone. I could not be alone even in my own house. I had to be with people because I was so afraid something terrible was going to happen to me when I was alone. So, I began staying at my parents' house when my husband worked the night shift. I was very lucky that my family was so understanding. They tried to help me as much as they could, which was very difficult to do because, at that point, I also had become quite paranoid.

If I had a headache, I was certain it was a brain tumor. When the headache ended, I would focus on some other physical ailment. If I had a pain in my calf, I just knew I had a blood clot. No one, not even a physician, could convince me I wasn't dying.

Finally, my cardiologist suggested I take a beta-blocker, and after just ten days on the medication, the panic attacks stopped. When I discontinued the beta-blocker, the panic attacks did not return. I haven't had a panic attack in fourteen years. If they ever returned, I would be more than willing to go back on that medication—or any other medication that my doctor recommended.

After I was relieved of the panic and paranoia, I felt capable of starting an exercise program, fluid loading, eliminating caffeine, and all the actions I needed to take to feel better. I had not realized how deconditioned I had become. It took me months of gradually building up to reach my optimal amount of exercise. Exercising regularly has proven very beneficial for me. It has brought my resting pulse down considerably, and I have much more energy than I used to have. Exercise also lowered my cholesterol.

Increasing my fluid intake helped to alleviate my fatigue, and it took away most of my dizziness. However, avoiding caffeine and sugar are still a real struggle. I'm a "chocoholic" and have been one for many years. I cannot avoid it completely, but I do know that when I eat chocolate, there will be a price to pay. I will get much more tired, and, in general, I'll just feel lousy.

So, how am I doing today, after finding out what I have, and after learning many coping skills and undergoing different treatments for the past fourteen years? Am I cured? Well, there is no cure. I do feel a whole lot better about myself. Actually, I feel like a completely different person.

I used to get so down on myself about my fears and phobias, and about not being "normal." The shame and guilt are tremendous when you want to do something and can't, or when you think you can't do something that other people do so easily and effortlessly, whether it be flying, driving, going out in crowds, and so forth. I learned not to "buy into" such shame and guilt anymore. I refuse to beat myself up any longer about anything.

The way I cope is by taking it one day at a time. I enjoy listening to motivational tapes. I love to play good, loud up-tempo music on days when I feel a little down. I try to stay away from negative people. My family has helped me overcome some of my fears. For example, I no longer have a medication phobia, so I am able to take the antidepressant I need for depression.

I do allow myself moments of self-pity. There are those days when I am not as positive and upbeat as I'd like to be. When that happens, I pity myself for a little while, and then I tell myself, "Now that's enough. It's time to move away from that and go back to being positive."

The life I lead now is the closest I've ever been to achieving the quality of life I want for myself. It's been a struggle, but it's getting much easier, and it is definitely worth it. I want other people with MVPS/D to learn what I have learned, so they, too, can live the type of life they wish for themselves. I hope to help as many people as I can through my work and my family's work with The Mitral Valve Prolapse Society.

Cheryl's story should bring hope to all of you with MVPS/D. She has made a lifetime commitment to modifying her lifestyle and continues to work on keeping her nervous system in balance to achieve the quality of life she wants for herself. Through education, determination, and diligence, Cheryl has become a success story.

Here is Jim's description of his lifetime struggle with MVPS/D:

Jim's Story

I've struggled with MVPS/D my whole life. As far back as I can remember I had symptoms like chest pains, palpitations, lightheadedness, fatigue, irritable bowel, severe anxiety, and phobias. I was able to live with most of these symptoms without them interfering too much in my life. My physical weakness and fatigue and the pounding and racing of my heart were everyday occurrences to me. They never scared me because I thought these were normal feelings that everyone else went through. On the other hand, irritable bowel was tough to deal with, physically as well as mentally. I don't know which was worse, worrying about having an attack of irritable bowel if I went out, or having an actual attack.

Anxiety was the one symptom that did severely interfere with my life. Anxiety was my worst enemy, living inside of me, directing and controlling my life. I was anxious pretty much most of the time, especially when engaging in new activities. It seemed that every month throughout my childhood I developed a new fear or phobia. I was scared of just about everything I thought could harm me: things like learning how to ride a bike and how to swim, as well as learning how to drive.

In fact, driving became my greatest phobia. My hands used to start sweating, even before I got in the car. Once I was in the driver's seat, my heart started pounding, my body started shaking, and my stomach started gurgling.

Some of my other phobias included using the telephone, being in social situations, making speeches, being alone at night, and being afraid of dogs.

I was always full of envy and amazement when I saw how others enjoyed taking part in the activities I feared. I was constantly asking myself, "Why am I different? Why am I not normal?" Most people looked at the fun or challenge that could result from trying something new. In most situations, I thought of what harm could come to me. After years of thinking this way, I developed what might be the worst fear of all—the fear of fear itself.

Years of anxiety took their toll on me, robbing me of my passions, as well as my self-esteem. I developed agoraphobia and avoided most activities outside of my home. My thinking became narrow-minded, that is, very focused on avoiding anxiety-provoking situations. Instead of going after life, I avoided it. My anxiety didn't allow me to look at or prepare for the future. Instead, it forced me to live day to day.

You'll be happy to know that I'm doing very well these days. Along with educating myself about MVPS/D, I had to also work on my self-esteem. Although it was difficult at first, changing my diet and starting to exercise regularly helped me immensely.

The most important thing I had to do to get better was to learn how to unlearn. For example, I had to unlearn some ridiculous lessons many children learn, especially male children. Lessons like, "Never admit you have problems, and if you do have problems, never ever talk about them." I had to unlearn thinking that anxiety, panic attacks, and depression are weaknesses. I also had to unlearn the stigma of going to a psychiatrist and taking medicine. It always amazes me how, for many people, the fear of talking about their problems can outweigh the problem itself.

> *Today, after everything I've been through, it is so gratifying to be part of The Mitral Valve Prolapse Society. I will continue to help others who have this disorder for as long as I possibly can.*

Jim has worked very hard at educating himself and learning how to get his nervous system back in balance. His is another success story. Jim, Cheryl, the authors of this book and their mother, Bonnie, have devoted much of their time to helping others with MVPS/D.

If you feel there are characteristics about yourself you need to change or would like to change, approach them slowly. If your life has been greatly affected in a negative way by MVPS/D, it did not happen overnight, and it will not change overnight. It will take time to turn things in a positive direction. When making changes, take baby steps. After all, you cannot walk before you crawl. Above all, don't ever believe that your problems are "all in your head."

MVPS/D is a real physiological syndrome, and you can learn to cope with it. It's not going to be easy, but it will be worth it. With hard work, persistence, and patience, you can change the balance of your nervous system. It is interesting to note here that people with MVPS/D are generally well-educated with an above average intelligence. They are also unusually creative and artistic (Rippetoe 1993). If these descriptors apply to you, they should help to put you on the road to recovery.

CHAPTER 6

Medical Diagnosis, Patient Advocacy, and Support Groups

A faithful friend is the medicine of life.

—Ecclesiastes 6:16

Today, people who once suffered silently from mitral valve prolapse syndrome/dysautonomia (MVPS/D) are beginning to speak up for themselves, their families, and for all those whose lives have been touched by this syndrome. As health care consumers, we are demanding more information, more involvement in making decisions about our care, and more effective treatments. These demands make good sense. After all, no one knows more about the state of our bodies and minds than we do.

Obtaining a Diagnosis

Before receiving a correct diagnosis, most people with MVPS/D have visited approximately ten physicians and endured numerous medical tests (Soffer 1999). Unfortunately, a diagnosis is not arrived at easily because there is no definitive test to determine whether or not someone has MVPS/D, and some physicians do not even believe that such a syndrome exists.

It's easier to obtain a diagnosis of MVPS/D if you already know that you have structural mitral valve prolapse, that is, the "floppy" valve. This is determined upon your physician hearing a "click" and/or murmur during a stethoscope examination or with a positive reading of your echocardiogram (see chapter 1).

If you have been diagnosed with structural mitral valve prolapse, your physician may then order a tilt-table test for you (see
chapter 2). This test is the most accurate way to determine the presence of MVPS/D. However, not all medical facilities have the capability to administer the tilt-table test. If this is the case, your
physician may take a prolonged standing test to determine the presence of MVPS/D (see chapter 2).

Also, because structural mitral valve prolapse has a genetic
component, be sure to inform your physician of any parents, sib-
lings, or other relatives who may have this defect. If your doctor sus-
pects that you have MVPS/D, but your test results are either
inconclusive or "borderline," he or she can make a clinical diagnosis
based on your symptoms or family history. Remember, both structural mitral valve prolapse (MVP) and MVPS/D tend to run in
families.

If you feel strongly that you exhibit the symptoms of MVPS/D,
but your echocardiogram is negative, and your physician does not
hear a click or murmur, you need to seek out a physician who is
open-minded and willing to listen to you. Remember, physicians are
required to treat symptoms, not test results.

Diagnostic Criteria

On July 1, 1999, *The New England Journal of Medicine* (Freed,
Levy, Levine, Larson, Evans, Fuller, et al. 1999) reported a study that
determined new criteria for diagnosing structural MVP. Although
some of the results of this study were encouraging, it did leave many
people confused.

The study involved 3,491 subjects, 1,845 of whom were women.
These participants ranged in age from twenty-six to eighty-four. All
of the subjects were given echocardiograms. In the past,
two-dimensional echocardiographic (M-mode) views were used to
diagnose MVP, but, of course, the valve itself is three-dimensional.

According to the study, in the past, this difference frequently
led some physicians to diagnose the presence of structural MVP in
normal subjects. Thus, you may have been diagnosed with structural
MVP many years ago, but that diagnosis may have been in error.
Today, because of new criteria for echocardiograph studies, you
might be told that you don't have MVP. Some people are being told
that they do have some kind of bulge or minor prolapse, but that it is
not significant enough to be classified as true structural MVP.

You may still have the syndrome, but you may be told now
that you don't have structural MVP. This is the reason that you

cannot rely solely on an echocardiogram to determine whether you have MVP. It is important to keep in mind that this study did not take the syndrome itself into consideration.

As Dr. Richard O. Russell, Jr., a cardiologist with Cardiovascular Associates, Inc., in Birmingham, Alabama, said at the 1993 Southwestern Conference on Mitral Valve Prolapse, "Diagnosis of dysautonomia (MVP syndrome) is a clinical diagnosis, not requiring the prolapse of the mitral valve to confirm or deny that diagnosis."

However, the diagnostic criteria have improved so much, that many fewer faulty diagnoses are being made. In the study cited in the 1999 article in *The New England Journal of Medicine* (Freed, Levy, Levine, Larson, Evans, Fuller, et al. 1999), two-dimensional echocardiography criteria *based on the three-dimensional saddlelike shape of the mitral valve were used.* After evaluating all of the subjects using these new criteria, it was found that only 2.4 percent of the subjects had MVP. These were surprising results when you consider that it had previously been believed that 4 to18 percent of the population has MVP. This study also verified the fact that people with MVP are not at a higher risk for heart disease and stroke than the normal population.

Educate Yourself

Educating yourself about MVPS/D is an important element of your treatment. By reading this book you have taken the first step toward that education. However, learning about this syndrome is no easy task. Unlike many other syndromes, there is not a great abundance of information out there.

One of the best ways to learn more about MVPS/D is to communicate with other people who have it. If you happen to be lucky enough to have a support group in your area, try to visit it. There's nothing like comparing notes with a group of people who are going through the same experiences that you are. If you can do this, you will quickly learn that everyone's stories are virtually the same as your own.

Refer to the Resources section in the back of this book to find MVPS/D information sources, such as newsletters, Web sites, videos, seminars, pen pals, and online chat groups. Be very careful when seeking information on the Internet. There is a lot of misinformation out there. Educating yourself about MVPS/D will be a continuous ongoing process, for life itself is an educational process. Knowledge is power—and also healing.

Support Groups

For people suffering from ills of all kinds, support groups provide emotional support and a place to share information. People dealing with such different medical issues as heart problems, cancer, and fibromyalgia all find acceptance and help in support groups. So, too, can those troubled by MVPS/D find help in support groups. But as the author of *The Fibromyalgia Advocate* put it:

> *Be careful.* There are some groups claiming to be support groups that are actually nothing more than "venting grounds." That is, the people in the group do little more than moan and groan about what a lousy hand life dealt them. A little venting is good for the soul and health of everyone. But if the entire discussion is focused on moaning and groaning, it will drag you down into the depths of negativity. *Avoid negative groups* (Starlanyl 1999, p. 72, emphasis in original).

If there is no group in your area, or if your only option is a group wallowing in negativity, think about starting a group of your own. You don't need more than a few people who meet to talk about how their lives are going and how they are managing to deal with the symptoms of MVPS/D. All the members can share information about coping skills and medications, and teach each other different affirmations and exercises.

> Whatever your needs are, you can be sure there are other people with the same needs. Find them. If there are a number of people who are interested in joining your support group, and you would like to use a public space to meet, many hospitals and public libraries offer meeting rooms at no charge or for a nominal fee (Starlanyl 1999, p. 72).

If you are interested in starting a support group, The Mitral Valve Prolapse Society (see Resources) will help you to start one. Besides helping yourself, you will be helping many others. A support group can be an extremely rewarding addition to your life.

You are not your illness. You are much more than that. Make sure you make the time to engage in activities totally unrelated to your MVPS/D. Whenever you can get away from it, do so. Remember, there are no limits on how much you can educate yourself. You can always learn more, think more deeply, and love more deeply.

Dealing with Your Physician

Unfortunately, when it comes to MVPS/D, you cannot rely on finding a good physician by specialty. Many people with MVPS/D think that they must be treated by a cardiologist. Although it is a good idea to get an initial diagnosis of structural MVP from a cardiologist, she or he is not necessarily the best physician to treat MVPS/D. Remember, it is an autonomic nervous system imbalance, not heart disease.

Of course, if you happen to be one of the rare people with *severe* structural MVP (see chapter 1), then a cardiologist is definitely the specialist who should be your treating physician. For most people with MVPS/D, however, the specialty of the physician is not as important as his or her ability to be compassionate and open-minded. Also, it is essential that you feel comfortable with your doctors and be able to talk to them as equals. Physicians who admit they really don't know much about MVPS/D sometimes turn out to be the best treating doctors around. They are honest and often feel comfortable learning about new medications or other treatments from their patients.

If you are happy with your current physician, that's great. If you aren't, you need to figure out why you aren't. Sometimes the reason isn't obvious. To help you figure out why you may not be happy with your doctor, ask yourself the following questions and write "yes" or "no" in the space provided. This checklist was adapted from *The Fibromyalgia Advocate* (2001) by Devin Starlanyl:

- Does your doctor pay attention when you are talking? Does she/he listen well, or keep looking at a clock? ____

- Does your doctor believe what you tell her or him? ____

- Do you have trust in your doctor's skill and knowledge? ____

- Do you feel it's okay to discuss all of your symptoms with your doctor? ____

- Do you ever think that your doctor hates to see your name on her/his calendar? ____

- Is your doctor's office staff polite to you on the phone and in the office? ____

- Is it hard or easy to make appointments? ____

- Does your doctor receive the phone messages you leave with the office staff? ____

- Are you encouraged to try new medications, or complementary medical treatments? ____

- Can you always ask questions and receive courteous answers? ____

- Will your doctor read information about MVPS/D that you bring to the office? ____

- Does your doctor do follow-up on tests, medications, and other treatments? ____

- Do you think that your doctor really cares about you? ____

If you answered "no" to five or more of these questions, it is very unlikely that you are being well-treated by your doctor.

Don't Be Afraid to Change Doctors

If your doctor is not providing you with what you need, which is quality care, perhaps it's time to change your doctor. You can ask people from your support group, your friends and relations, and your church and club members whether they can recommend a good doctor for you. You need a doctor who can help you find what you need to feel better. You deserve to feel as well as you possibly can.

Have you ever heard the following (or something like it) from your physician? "Mitral valve prolapse is a benign condition. It means nothing. Just go home and forget about it." Or, "All your tests come back negative. There's nothing wrong with you. You're lucky to be so healthy." If these are the types of statements you have heard, then it is definitely time for you to find a new doctor for yourself.

You and Your Dentist

If you have been diagnosed with MVP, be sure to inform your dentist of this. Mitral valve prolapse and leakage (regurgitation) put you at a slightly greater risk for contracting endocarditis than the rest of the population. You may need to take antibiotics when you are undergoing dental treatments to prevent endocarditis.

The American Heart Association (AHA) recommends antibiotic treatments for patients with prolapsing and leaking mitral valves that have been evidenced by audible clicks or murmurs, either upon stethoscope examination or by evidence from a color Doppler (Dajani, Taubert, Wilson, Bolger, Bayer, Ferrieri, et al. 1997). The Doppler technique adds color to an echocardiogram. This helps to reveal how the blood is flowing from the heart through its four valves. It demonstrates any disturbances to the normal flow of blood, such as regurgitation, that is, when the blood flow is backwards (see chapter 1) and stenosis, that is, the constriction or narrowing of an opening.

A course of antibiotic treatment is also recommended for patients whose mitral leaflets appear to have thickened as shown on an echocardiogram. For men who are forty-five or older with MVP, but with no consistent systolic murmur, it may be wise to take antibiotics when receiving dental care, even though no regurgitation was noted during a resting heart examination (Dajani, Taubert, Wilson, Bolger, Bayer, Ferrieri, et al. 1997). It is essential that you check with your dentist and your physician before having dental procedures to see whether you should take antibiotics. The American Heart Association (1997) recommended antibiotics for people who have MVP for the following dental procedures:

- Extractions

- Periodontal procedures

- Dental implant placements

- Root canal treatments

- Placement of antibiotic fibers or strips subgingivally (below the gums)

- Initial placement of orthodontic bands, but not brackets

- Cleaning of teeth or implants where bleeding is anticipated

Also, ask your dentist about a local anesthesia with 3-percent carbacaine, because it contains no epinephrine (adrenaline). Novocaine may cause you to experience tachycardia, palpitations, and anxiety if you are prone to suffering from these symptoms.

You and Your Pharmacist

Imagine this scene: Your physician has just prescribed a beta-blocker for you; now you're at the pharmacy waiting to have your prescription filled. You can't remember everything your physician told you, and questions are swimming in your head. "When should I start taking this? Is it all right to take this prescription with the one I'm taking for anxiety? Are there any side effects? How often should I take this?"

The person who can knowledgeably answer questions like these is your pharmacist. Although pharmacists cannot diagnose illnesses, they are doing more and more to help patients. For example, computers now enable pharmacists to keep tabs on which medications you are currently taking, so they can alert you if you are taking medications that interact poorly with each other.

Fortunately, recent legislation requiring pharmacists to counsel customers about their medications has given consumers unprecedented access to their pharmacists' expertise. If you find it difficult to talk to your pharmacist privately when in the drugstore, feel free to call. Most pharmacists welcome phone consultations. A good pharmacy is one that serves your needs.

Health Insurance

Today, the entire practice of medicine is in transition. The days of the general practitioner who made house calls at all hours of the night are long gone. This is the era of specialists, high-tech diagnostic aids, and managed health care, where the insurance companies, not the doctors, have the final say about treatments.

In this new millenium, we are seeing people with MVPS/D turned down for health insurance every day. This is the unfortunate result of past shortcomings in diagnosis and treatment. In the past, people with the multiple symptoms of MVPS/D were subjected to great numbers of diagnostic procedures, emergency room visits, and hospital admissions, as well as numerous visits to assorted specialists. The costs added up, and the people who run the insurance companies concluded that those patients who had structural MVP were more expensive to care for than patients who had other disorders.

People with MVP are often either turned down entirely for insurance coverage or they can receive only limited coverage, with a waiver attached. Depending on what type of waiver it is, it will generally state that the insurance company will not cover anything having to do with mitral valve prolapse for anywhere from two to ten years from the time the policy is issued.

If you are having difficulty getting health insurance because of having MVP, you can sometimes receive coverage by including a letter from your doctor with your application. Fortunately, it now seems as if more and more insurance companies are beginning to understand that mitral valve prolapse is a benign condition.

People with MVP used to be categorized under the overall umbrella of heart disease, and the medical profession has not done a good job of educating the insurance industry. Some hidebound insurance companies still classify MVP as heart disease. Their underwriters have no idea what MVP or MVPS/D are all about. Such companies are the ones who can make life very difficult for people with either condition.

For example, here is Sandra's account of her difficulties in obtaining health insurance:

> *After going through a traumatic divorce, I also had to deal with losing the health insurance coverage I had had through my ex-husband's employer. I applied for and was denied health insurance by three different insurance companies because I have MVP.*
>
> *I wrote several letters to these companies explaining that my MVP was a benign condition, but it was not until my doctor wrote a letter to an insurance company on my behalf explaining that my heart function was perfectly normal, that I finally received coverage.*

However, there was a waiver attached to her policy stating that she would not be covered for anything pertaining to MVP for the next five years. Sandra accepted that coverage, but she is still applying to other companies to see if she can obtain health insurance without a waiver attached that denies her treatment for her specific condition.

If you have been turned down by an insurance company, don't give up. As Sandra's story illustrates, it is sometimes helpful to have your physician write a letter to the company stating that your heart function is normal. Now, since the 1999 study reported in *The New England Journal of Medicine* (Freed, Levy, Levine, Larson, Evans, Fuller, et al. 1999) demonstrated that people with MVP are not at a higher risk for heart disease or stroke, matters are slowly beginning to change in the insurance industry.

Your Right to Your Medical Records

Devin Starlanyl discussed your right to your medical records in her book, *The Fibromyalgia Advocate* (1999). I cannot improve upon her discussion, so here's what she had to say:

> The right to obtain your medical records varies from state to state. The original records belong to your physician, but,

in most cases, you have the right to obtain an exact copy. Don't expect to get the originals. Your physician needs those for legal documentation. Contact your local representative in the State Legislature of your state, and ask for information on how to get copies of your patient records.

If you want to obtain your mental health records, as well, be sure to specify that, because many states differentiate between patient records and patient mental health records. If you have been refused access to your records, explain that to the state representative. Be as brief and concise as possible when speaking to the representative. Be sure to give the representative names, addresses, and phone numbers. Make it easy for others to help you. Follow up your original inquiries to make sure that any promises made to you are kept (p. 196).

You can file a legal complaint about a doctor by getting in touch with the State Board of Medicine in your state. Usually, the Board has been mandated by state law to investigate all complaints. As a rule, you can obtain the forms you need from the Board by writing and asking for them. Be sure to include a stamped, self-addressed envelope with your request for the complaint forms.

To report your complaint to the State Medical Board, you must provide them with the name, address, and phone number of your doctor. You will also need to give them your name, and the name of the patient, if you are not the patient (e.g., if you are the patient's spouse, child, or parent). The Board will need to know the dates of all of your appointments and treatments, as well as any other pertinent information about your complaint.

Send *copies* of any supporting documents with your complaint form. Do not send the originals. The Board will send you a "Release of Information" form. If you are worried about your doctor learning about your complaint while you are still under her/his care, try calling the Board instead of writing. You may feel more at ease expressing your doubts and worries about the doctor over the phone. The complaint form usually has the telephone number you will need printed on the cover page.

Your Obligations to Your Doctor

If you have a good doctor, you are very fortunate. Do what you can to retain him or her. After a few years of treating you, your primary care doctor has a lot more information about you than just what's in your medical folder. That information may be very useful to you in years to come. So, if you have a good doctor, you want to continue to maintain good relations with him or her. Understanding your obligations to your health providers goes a long way toward creating and maintaining beneficial relationships with them. Here are some of your obligations:

- Come prepared to the doctor's office. Bring whatever relevant notes you have made.

- Don't announce that you have just diagnosed what ails you. You are going to the doctor to learn what he or she thinks about your condition.

- Do not lie to your doctor about anything.

- Stay on topic during the length of your office visit.

- Don't cancel appointments except for dire emergencies.

- Be on time for all appointments.

- Be sure to inform your doctor of all the medications you may be taking. This includes over-the-counter medications.

- Pay your bills on time. If you cannot pay all that you owe, discuss time payments with your doctor.

- It has been many years since doctors were on call twenty-four hours a day, so be sure to respect your doctor's needs for rest and relaxation.

Support from Family and Friends

Your family and friends can be a critical factor in helping you to cope with your MVPS/D. They can provide emotional support, caring, and guidance. A great way for your family and friends to help you is by learning as much as they possibly can about MVPS/D and its treatment by reading books or attending conferences and support group meetings. They may have unnecessary worries if they don't know the facts about MVPS/D. If they understand the syndrome better, they can better provide you with support and understanding.

Asking for Help

As you learn to live with MVPS/D, you may feel a greater need to call on your family and friends for help. There may be times when you need help cleaning the house, getting places, taking care of your children, buying groceries, or accomplishing other tasks. You'd like to be able to do all of these things yourself, but you have to realize it just may not be possible when your MVPS/D symptoms are bothering you.

Don't think that you must do everything yourself. There's nothing wrong with reaching out for help. Asking for help is certainly a better choice than pushing yourself beyond your limits, and suffering the consequences later. The likelihood is good that your family and/or your friends will want to pitch in and help you when help is needed. Sometimes, all that is needed is making that first request.

Changing Your Plans

It is difficult having to change plans with friends at the last minute because you're so fatigued that you can't even move. You can understand how your friends might feel if this happens frequently. Good friends who understand, or at least try to understand, what you're going through probably will be able to accept these changes. Others may be less willing to put up with them.

For example, Kathy hated it when she and her husband made plans with friends, and she had to bow out because of her MVPS/D symptoms. She had to stay home alone because no one else wanted to change their plans. Since problems like this can be an unfortunate part of living with MVPS/D, discussing these issues with your family and friends can only help, and may result in increased tolerance and understanding that will maintain good relationships.

Spending Time with Your Children

One of the hardest parts of dealing with your children may be dealing with their disappointment when you can't do everything with them that they'd like to do. You want to spend a lot of time with your children, taking them places, and doing things with them. If this doesn't happen, you may feel guilty, but let's face it, having MVPS/D can be very restrictive. The fatigue, especially, may prevent you from doing a lot of what you'd like to do.

You may need to explain to your children that you're not able to do as much as you'd like to do. You can try to come to an agreement with them about an enjoyable activity you can do together, when you're feeling better. Making such arrangements will show your children that you're aware of their feelings and lets them know that you want to spend time with them, even when you can't.

Denial

What should you do if your family and friends simply won't accept the fact that you have MVPS/D? You might hear things like, "Come on. You look fine. What are you complaining about?" You can try to educate them, but don't go overboard. Constantly talking about MVPS/D all the time will not make them change their minds. They will accept the fact that you have MVPS/D when they are ready.

Tips for Family Members

- If your loved one is undergoing therapy, see that the doctor's orders are followed. Encourage him or her to stick to the doctor's recommendations. Any medications should be taken exactly as the doctor instructed them to be taken.

- Keep the person separate from MVPS/D. Love the person even if you hate the MVPS/D.

- It's *not* okay for you to neglect yourself if you are helping the person with MVPS/D. It's important for family members and friends to take care of themselves, too.

- A family member or a friend who has MVPS/D is nothing to be ashamed of. Remind him or her that deciding to do something about MVPS/D and its symptoms is very courageous. Tell him or her that you support whatever actions are needed to alleviate the symptoms.

- Remember, no one is to blame.

- It's natural and acceptable to feel a mix of emotions such as guilt, fear, anger, and sadness. It may be as hard for the person with MVPS/D to accept it as it is for family and friends.

- Learn all you can about MVPS/D.

- You and your family are not alone. Sharing your thoughts and feelings with friends or a support group can be very helpful.

- Be patient. This is a long journey with many ups and downs.

- Encourage your loved one to do his or her best every day.

Don't Use MVPS/D as an Excuse

As you know by now, the symptoms of MVPS/D can be debilitating, especially if left untreated. There are going to be times when you need to push yourself to get certain tasks accomplished. Conversely, you may be tempted occasionally to use your symptoms as an excuse.

For example, if you really don't want to go somewhere, but you feel you are obliged to attend, you might say that you have a migraine headache or that you are too fatigued. This is not a good idea. As a patient advocate, it is important for you to spread the word about MVPS/D in a legitimate fashion. As lay people and the medical profession begin to understand that this is indeed a true syndrome, more research will be done and, therefore, more questions about MVPS/D will be answered. In the meantime, it will not help your cause if you use your illness to cover up your absences from events that you really did not want to attend.

Furthermore, although your physicians play an important role in helping you to cope with MVPS/D, don't rely on them totally to restore your autonomic nervous system to a normally functioning state. Ultimately, how you deal with this syndrome is up to you.

Once you do everything in your power that you need to do to get your nervous system back in balance, hopefully, you will want to become an advocate and help to spread the word about MVPS/D. It is quite gratifying to teach others what you have learned, and you will be rewarded for it in more ways than you can imagine.

CHAPTER 7

Nutrition

Tell me what you eat, and I'll tell you what you are.

—Anthelme Brillat-Savarin

For those who have mitral valve prolapse/dysautonomia (MVPS/D), there are special dietary considerations that should be observed. That's because people with MVPS/D often tend to have very low energy levels, and an inadequate diet can further aggravate this problem, as well as many other symptoms. Therefore, if you have MVPS/D, it is extremely important for you to follow a nutritionally complete, well-balanced diet as part of your treatment.

Fluid Loading

Some of the symptoms of MVPS/D such as dizziness, lightheadedness, and feeling faint, are due to low blood pressure and low circulating blood volume. Many people with MVPS/D are *hypovolemic*, which means that your body may have 80 to 85 percent of the blood volume, or fluid, it is supposed to have, as was previously discussed in chapter 2 (Roach 1998).

In order to maintain adequate blood volume, you must get into the habit of fluid loading so that you will stay hydrated. The importance of fluid loading cannot be stressed too strongly because dehydration, even when mild, can cause tachycardia and fatigue. As stated in chapter 3 you should drink eight eight-ounce glasses of fluid per day. That's 64 ounces of fluid. When it is warmer outside, drink one ounce of fluid for each degree of the outside temperature. For example, if it is 80 degrees outside, you should drink 80 ounces of nonalcoholic fluid.

Furthermore, if you exercise vigorously, particularly in outdoor sports, you should also fluid load. Ski trips or other excursions to high altitudes can cause symptoms to start up very abruptly. The dehydrating effects of altitude and long-distance plane travel tend to aggravate these symptoms. Therefore, it is extremely important for you to fluid load before and during a trip.

Your primary fluid should be water, although a noncaffeine-containing drink will suffice. Some of the sports drinks, such as Gatorade, contain electrolytes, which are important for maintaining the proper body fluid level. You will have to be vigilant about your fluid intake, because you may not be very thirsty throughout the day.

It seems that people with MVPS/D may have an inadequate thirst mechanism (Watkins 1990). You might have to learn how to fluid load by actually forcing yourself to drink more often. As you increase your fluid intake, fluid loading will soon become a habit, and you will find it is a beneficial aspect of your treatment.

Salt and Low Blood Pressure

For the past decade it has been believed that salt is bad for you. As far as MVPS/D is concerned, currently it appears that salt is harmful only to the small percentage of people with this syndrome who have high blood pressure. If you have high blood pressure, it would probably be prudent to limit your salt intake.

Most people with MVPS/D, however, tend to have rather low blood pressure, although there are, of course, exceptions (MVP Center 1993). If you are one of those who have very low blood pressure, you should keep your salt intake at normal to high levels. If your intake is limited dramatically you may feel much worse because your blood pressure will drop even further. When this happens it may cause you to feel faint, lightheaded, and/or dizzy.

If you think you need to increase your salt intake, you can start by snacking on pretzels and by using salt to season your food. Of course, any important decision about changing your diet should first be discussed with your physician, and increasing your salt intake is definitely one such important decision. The following table provides you with a handy reference to check the amount of salt you consume (Rowe, Calkins, and Kan 2002). It would be a good idea for you to get some notion of what your daily salt intake is so that you will know whether you consume under or over the recommended amount. The FDA-recommended daily amount of salt is under 2400 milligrams (2.4 grams). One gram is composed of 1,000 milligrams (Sacher 2000).

Salt Amount Per Serving Size of Food

Food	Serving Size	Milligrams of Sodium
Gatorade	1 cup	110
Wheaties	1 cup	500
Waffles	1	400
All Bran	1/2 cup	355
Cheerios	1 cup	285
Rice Krispies	1 cup	260
Saltine crackers	6	200
Parmesan cheese	1 ounce	450
Cottage cheese	1/2 cup	230
Processed cheese	1 ounce	320
Cheese spreads	1 ounce	320
Dill pickle	1	1430
Tomato juice	8 ounces	800
Sweet pickle	1	570
Canned vegetables	1/2 cup	245
Canned tomato sauce/puree	1/4 cup	370
Frozen vegetables w/sauce	1/2 cup	375
TV dinner	1	1300
Sweet and sour pork	1 serving	1200
Lasagna	1 serving	1100
Soup, canned	1 cup	895
Fish and chips	1 serving	750
Hamburger	1	690
Hot dog	1	550

Tuna, canned	1/2 cup	535
Pizza, cheese	1 slice	500
Luncheon meat	1 slice	300
Bacon	4 slices	280
Soy sauce	1 tablespoon	870
Olives, green	4	600
Salted nuts	1/2 cup	420
Olives, ripe	4	400
Fruit pie	1/8 pie serving	355

Recommendations for a Heart-Healthy Diet

Your mind and your body are made from the food you eat. There-fore, they are dependent on good nutrition to maintain optimal health and functionality. Choosing proper foods is one of your best defenses against heart disease. Good nutrition may also be helpful in preventing many types of cancer which, next to heart disease, is the number one killer in our nation. Of course, a heart-healthy diet is recommended for people with MVPS/D and everyone else, as well.

A 2000 American Heart Association conference document (Sacher 2000) reviewed strategies for maintaining a heart-healthy diet. Many experts recommended the following as generally accepted standards for what people should eat every day:

- Less than 10 percent of your total daily calories should come from saturated fat.

- Less than 10 percent of your total daily calories should come from polyunsaturated fat.

- Less than 10 percent of your total daily calories should come from monounsaturated fat.

- Less than 30 percent of your total daily calories should come from any type of fat.

- More than 55 percent of your total daily calories should come from complex carbohydrates (starches).

- Your total cholesterol intake should be under 300 milligrams daily.

People with MVPS/D should never consume less than 1200 calories per day (MVP Center 1987). A number of smaller meals throughout the day can enhance your level of energy. Because your energy levels will be lower in the morning, start your day with a nutritious breakfast to provide your body with an adequate fuel supply.

Cholesterol and Fats

There are three types of fats: saturated, monounsaturated, and polyunsaturated. All have the same number of calories, yet they affect your blood cholesterol levels differently. Cholesterol is *not* a fat. It is a waxy, fat-like substance produced by all human beings. Cholesterol is needed for many bodily functions and serves to insulate nerve fibers, maintain cell walls, and produce vitamin D, various hormones, and digestive juices. Cholesterol is manufactured by your liver.

Blood cholesterol can be broken down into two major parts: HDL, or high-density lipoprotein and LDL, or low-density lipoprotein. The HDL is known as "good cholesterol" because it helps to move cholesterol back to the liver for removal from the bloodstream. The LDL is known as "bad cholesterol" because it can adhere to artery walls.

Saturated fat raises blood cholesterol and LDL levels more than any other element in your diet. It is the predominant fat in animal foods. Palm oil, coconut oil, and cocoa butter contain large amounts of saturated fat.

Monounsaturated and polyunsaturated fats may actually lower your blood cholesterol levels when they replace saturated fat in your diet. Foods rich in monounsaturated fat include olive oil, canola oil, and nuts. High levels of polyunsaturated fat are found in most cooking oils.

Reducing your saturated fat intake may result in lowering your cholesterol consumption, because many high-fat foods are also rich in cholesterol. It is equally important to cut back on your total fat intake. Luckily, the two go hand in hand, since most low-fat foods are also low in saturated fat.

You do not have to consume low-fat and low-cholesterol food exclusively. You should practice moderation by balancing foods high in fat or cholesterol with low-fat selections.

Red Meat

We hear all the time that we should consume less red meat, yet there is more cholesterol in the white meat of chicken than there is in beef or pork. So what should we be eating? Although it is true that there is more cholesterol in the white meat from chicken than in most other lean cuts of beef and pork, a food's total fat grams and saturated fat grams have a greater impact on your blood cholesterol level and your risk for heart disease. There is more total fat and saturated fat in beef and pork than there is in a chicken breast.

It is important that you eat a variety of foods, including meat, poultry, fish, and even vegetarian meals. When you take this variety of food into consideration, cholesterol and fat intakes average out over time. This does not mean you should forget about the cholesterol and fat content of the foods you eat. When it comes to eating poultry, beef, pork, or even fish, it is important to remember to keep your intake to no more than five to six ounces daily. Furthermore, be sure you select the leanest grades (choice or select) and the leanest cuts (loin, sirloin, or round).

As far as food preparation is concerned, you should trim away the fat of beef or pork cuts before preparing, and remove the skin of poultry before eating. Cook your meat without fat and in such a way that the fat in the meat melts and drips away, such as baking or grilling. This will ensure that more fat isn't added, and that the fat that is naturally in the food is minimized.

Eggs and Dairy Products

Whoever said "moderation in all things," must have had nutrition in mind. A healthful diet does not exclude any one food or food group. Moreover, it may include your favorite foods. The best diet is based on breads, grains, cereals, fruits, and vegetables that are rich in complex carbohydrates and fiber, low in fat, and full of vitamins and minerals. A balanced diet also includes high-protein foods like eggs and low-fat dairy products.

Eggs and dairy products are loaded with key vitamins and minerals. Eggs are also rich in protein and low in sodium. There is no need for you to totally avoid eggs on a heart-healthy diet. Many cholesterol-lowering diets do allow moderate amounts of whole eggs. Of course, there is no limit on egg whites, since they're both cholesterol- and fat-free. To reduce fat intake, poach your eggs instead of frying them, and use nonstick pans or nonstick vegetable pan spray when preparing eggs.

As for dairy products, switching from butter to soft and liquid margarine, such as Benecol, from whole or 2-percent milk to 1-percent or skim milk, and choosing the lighter varieties of dairy products, such as cheese made with nonfat or low-fat milk, fat-free or low-fat yogurt, and fat-free or low-fat ice cream, reduces your risk for heart disease.

Alcohol

There is no absolute contraindication to consuming alcohol if you have MVPS/D. However, people with MVPS/D do have a sensitive nervous system, and they tend to react to alcohol in an exaggerated fashion. Many people have reported to us that they are unable to drink even small amounts of alcohol because it makes their symptoms worse.

If you are on antidepressants or anti-anxiety medications, be sure to check with your physician about the safety of drinking, and the possible interaction of your medication and alcohol. If you do drink occasionally, make sure to drink only moderate amounts.

How Alcohol Affects the Autonomic Nervous System

Alcohol is a central nervous system depressant. It depresses your breathing rate and your heart rate. The effects of this depression on your central nervous system may include the following:

- Impaired ability to perform complex tasks, such as driving

- Reduction of inhibitions

- Reduction in anxiety

- Decreased attention span

- Impaired short-term memory

- Impaired motor coordination

- Prolonged reaction times

- Slower thought processing

Some people with MVPS/D are tempted to drink alcohol because it will reduce their anxiety. However, drinking will only give you short-term relief. In the long run, drinking alcohol to reduce your anxiety will be detrimental to your MVPS/D symptoms, your lifestyle, and your health in general.

How Alcohol Causes Dehydration

Alcohol has a diuretic effect on the body. The more alcohol you consume, the more water loss you will experience, and this may lead to dehydration. The degree of dehydration depends on how much water you consume with the alcohol. The greater your water intake, the less the dehydration. Keep in mind that drinking water protects against dehydration, not against intoxication.

How Alcohol Causes Palpitations and Tachycardia

Alcohol in small amounts can be a stimulant. Stimulation of your nervous system can cause palpitations and tachycardia. Also, if you become dehydrated from drinking alcohol, you may find that you will experience palpitations and/or tachycardia.

How Alcohol Triggers IBS Symptoms

People with MVPS/D find that different foods and beverages aggravate their irritable bowel syndrome (IBS) symptoms. For some people, alcohol may aggravate IBS symptoms. For instance, if the form your IBS takes is predominantly diarrhea, it is best to avoid alcohol entirely. Keeping a diary of your food and beverage intake may help you find out what things activate your IBS symptoms and should therefore be avoided.

How Alcohol Causes Insomnia

Alcohol consumed at bedtime, after its initial stimulating effect, may decrease the time required to fall asleep. Because of alcohol's sedating effect, many people with insomnia consume alcohol to promote sleep. However, alcohol consumed within an hour of bedtime appears also to disrupt sleep. That is, the person with insomnia may fall asleep more quickly after a drink or two, but his or her sleep will most likely be interrupted by wakefulness one or more times during the night. Such sleep disruption may lead to greater daytime fatigue and sleepiness.

Alcoholic beverages are often consumed in the late afternoon at "happy hour" or with dinner without further consumption before bedtime. But a moderate amount of alcohol consumed as long as six hours before bedtime can increase wakefulness. By the time this wakefulness effect occurs, the dose of alcohol consumed that afternoon has already been eliminated from the body. This suggests that a relatively long-lasting change has occurred in the body's mechanisms for regulating sleep.

Red Wine's Effect on the Heart

Red wine may suppress one of the main chemical culprits thought to cause heart disease. A new study has found that red wine blocks a cellular compound thought to be a key factor in heart disease, thus bolstering claims that red wine carries more health benefits than other alcoholic beverages (Corder, Douthwaite, Lees, Khan, Viseu dos Santos, Wood, et al. 2001). The study suggests that nonalcoholic extracts from red wine inhibit the formation of endothelin-1, a chemical that causes blood vessels to constrict. Compounds that block endothelin-1 may reduce the formation of fatty streaks in blood vessels and thus decrease heart attack risk.

White and rosé wines had no effect on the production of endothelin-1. This implies that the active ingredients are polyphenols, which are compounds from grape skins found only in red wines. This finding may help explain why the French, who often drink red wine with their meals, appear to have a lower risk of heart disease than people in other countries, despite their eating a similar amount of saturated fat. This is a phenomenon known as the "French paradox."

Sugar and Caffeine

Both sugar and caffeine can stimulate the autonomic nervous system, thus causing your symptoms of MVPS/D to become more pronounced. Therefore, eliminating caffeine from your diet and reducing your intake of refined sugars (as opposed to natural sugars such as those in fruit) can be a very positive step toward controlling your symptoms.

Sugar and Caffeine: Two Dangerous Nutritional "Culprits"

Sugar and MVPS/D are a terrible combination. Although you may feel a boost of quick energy after eating something sweet, approximately thirty minutes later you will more than likely feel worse than you did before you ate the sugar.

To understand why this happens, follow the sequence of physical events that take place when you put large amounts of sugar into your body in a short period of time. Suppose you eat a chocolate candy bar because you feel the need for some quick energy. Here is what happens inside your body:

- Sugar is absorbed rapidly from your digestive tract into your bloodstream.

- To clear the sugar from your bloodstream and to help your cells absorb that sugar to produce energy, insulin is secreted from your pancreas. Immediately following this, the boost of energy takes place.

- Insulin causes your blood sugar levels to fall too low.

- When blood sugar levels drop significantly, your brain is rapidly deprived of energy.

- Adrenal glands release adrenaline to protect your brain.

- Such a release of adrenaline can cause chronic fatigue, heart palpitations, a rapid heartbeat, and anxiety.

If, at this point, you eat another piece of chocolate either to boost your energy again, or for comfort, you will start the entire cycle over again. The only way to break this cycle is to replace the sugar-laden foods with a nutritious, high-protein snack such as cheese, or peanut butter and crackers. It's a good idea to eat a high-protein snack mid-morning and mid-afternoon.

Caffeine may be even worse for those with MVPS/D than sugar is. Caffeine is a drug that stimulates adrenaline production which, in turn, raises blood sugar levels. The high blood sugar level then makes the pancreas overwork by sending out erratic, or excessive, amounts of insulin, alternately raising and lowering blood sugar levels. This explains the boost of energy followed by a "let-down," or the "high-low" symptom that so many of us complain about.

Caffeine stimulates your sympathetic nervous system, increasing your heart rate and your blood pressure at rest, and causing arrhythmias. It causes other adverse effects which are related to the central nervous system. These adverse effects include restlessness, hyperactivity, irritability, dry mouth, insomnia, and depression.

If you try to limit your caffeine intake drastically, you may experience severe headaches. Caffeine should be removed from your diet gradually. You can taper off your caffeine intake by cutting your consumption in half for one week, then cut it in half again, and then cut out caffeine completely. This gradual approach seems to prevent the headache response. If you remove caffeine from your diet you will experience a great deal more energy and avoid its destabilizing effect on your autonomic nervous system.

Caffeine Content in Favorite Foods

Food	Serving Size	Milligrams of Caffeine
Coffee, brewed	8 ounces	135
Coffee, instant	8 ounces	95
Tea, leaf or bag	8 ounces	50
Lipton tea	8 ounces	35-40
Snapple iced tea	16 ounces	42
Tea, green	8 ounces	30
Tea, instant	8 ounces	15
Mountain Dew	12 ounces	55 1/2
Diet Coke	12 ounces	46 1/2
Coke	12 ounces	34 1/2
Dr. Pepper, regular or Diet	12 ounces	42
Pepsi	12 ounces	37 1/2
Sprite or Diet Sprite	12 ounces	0
7-Up, Regular or Diet	12 ounces	0
Barq's root beer	12 ounces	0
Hershey Bar, milk chocolate	1 bar	10
Cocoa or hot chocolate	8 ounces	5
Starbucks coffee ice cream	1 cup	40–60
Dannon coffee yogurt	8 ounces	45

Changing Your Diet

Dietary habits can be difficult to change. This is well-known to those of you who have attempted dieting for weight control. You begin a calorie control program and do very well for a few weeks, but soon you return to your old habits and you watch your weight quickly return—and then some.

The recommendations for dietary modifications are quite simple to list, but much more difficult to implement. However, if you make these changes for several weeks and notice improvements in your MVPS/D symptoms, you will find it easier to incorporate these dietary changes into your permanent treatment plan.

Motivation

Maintaining a healthy body weight is one of the best things you can do to ensure good health. Lugging around extra fat, especially fat around the abdomen, increases your chances for heart disease, diabetes, and high blood pressure. It may also aggravate lower back pain and contribute to low energy levels.

Many people exercise for weight control. But regular exercise can do much more than help you to lose weight or maintain weight loss: Regular exercise preserves and builds muscle and bone tissue, increases flexibility, improves the body's response to insulin, and helps control blood pressure. In addition, physical activity may lower blood cholesterol levels and increase levels of HDL, the desirable cholesterol. The higher your HDL, the better. More to the point, it appears that active people live longer than sedentary types.

Diets and Weight

Successful weight loss and healthy weight management depend on sensible goals and expectations. If you set sensible goals for yourself, chances are you will be more likely to meet them and you will have a better chance of keeping the weight off.

If you are overweight, you should lose weight gradually. For safe and healthy weight loss, try not to lose more than two pounds per week. Exceeding this rate may cause you also to lose water and muscle, which may lead to fatigue and a worsening of your MVPS/D symptoms. Sometimes, people with serious health problems associated with obesity may have legitimate reasons for losing weight rapidly. If this is true in your case, a physician's supervision is essential.

What you weigh is the result of a combination of the following several factors:

- Your diet, including how much and what kinds of food you eat

- Your lifestyle and whether it includes regular physical activity

- Your use of food to respond to stress and other situations in your life

- Your physiologic and genetic make-up

- Your age and health status

Successful weight loss and weight management should address all of these factors. That's the reason you should ignore products and programs that promise quick and easy results, or that promise permanent results without permanent changes in your lifestyle. Any ad that says you can lose weight without lowering your caloric intake and/or increasing your physical activity is selling fantasy and false hope. In fact, some people call it fraud. Furthermore, the use of some of the products that use these kinds of ads may not be safe.

For example, appetite suppressants, or diet pills, reduce your appetite by way of stimulation of the sympathetic nervous system. The problem with them is the frequency and severity of their side effects. Diet pills can cause anxiety, depression, insomnia, irritability, delusions, elevation of blood pressure, rapid heart rate, palpitations, headaches, and gastrointestinal disturbances. Furthermore, tolerance to diet pills develops rapidly, usually within weeks, thus making them ineffective for long-term use. For these reasons they are not recommended for someone who needs to lose ten to fifteen pounds, but rather only for the seriously obese person, and only then under a physician's supervision.

Since the majority of people with MVPS/D already experience significant overactivity of the sympathetic nervous system, they will almost certainly experience serious side effects if they use these pills. Therefore, diet pills are contraindicated for anyone with MVPS/D.

Fad diets may result in short-term weight loss, but they may do so at the risk of your health. How you go about managing your weight has a lot to do with your long-term success. Unless your health is seriously at risk because of complications from being obese, gradual weight loss should be your rule—and your goal.

Food Allergies and Sensitivities

Symptoms of food allergies, intolerances, and sensitivities can be amplified and worsened by MVPS/D. These symptoms include feeling spaced out, inability to concentrate, digestive upset, and fatigue.

Many people are sensitive to such common foods as milk, wheat, corn, and nuts without realizing it. They have been eating these foods for so long and so frequently that they don't make the connection between them and their symptoms. Adverse reactions to food can be very hard to pin down since they can occur instantly or several hours after the ingestion of a particular food. Some foods can trigger a whole range of symptoms, and these symptoms can wax and wane in their severity. Some food allergies worsen during times of great stress, or they can be seasonal.

The one surefire way to find out whether you're allergic, intolerant, or sensitive to a food is to eliminate it from your diet. After four days, reintroduce it under the supervision of your physician. At the end of the four-day abstinence from that food, when it is reintroduced to your body, your symptoms may reappear in a marked and obvious manner. There will then be no doubt about whether you are allergic or not.

An "elimination diet" is highly effective and should be overseen by your doctor. You need to be monitored carefully. In many cases, the food should be reintroduced in small amounts, as little as half a teaspoon, to prevent highly unpleasant reactions.

The need to modify your lifestyle in order to control the symptoms of MVPS/D cannot be overstressed. Too often in our fast-paced culture we seek quick answers and instant cures. Nowhere is this more common than when dealing with MVPS/D. If you seek to control it with the use of medications alone you will surely fail. Make the commitment today that you will begin to make the needed changes that will maximize your chances of living a healthy lifestyle.

CHAPTER 8

Fatigue and Sleep Problems

Fatigue is when your mind says yes, but your body says no.

—Anonymous

Fatigue is the feeling of extreme tiredness or exhaustion, often involving muscle weakness, that can result in difficulties when performing even very simple tasks. It has been compared to the tired and achy feeling you have when you have the flu; however, fatigue can last longer and recur more often. Fatigue is one of the most common symptoms reported by people with mitral valve prolapse syndrome/dysautonomia (MVPS/D). In a study of almost 2,000 patients with MVPS/D 92 percent reported fatigue as their most common complaint (Watkins 1997).

In some cases, you'll feel tired following an activity or some expenditure of energy. In other cases, fatigue arrives out of the blue, it comes as a total surprise. You may not have done anything tiring, when all of a sudden, fatigue can hit your body like a ton of bricks. You can feel as if the energy has drained right out of your body. It seems impossible for you to do anything at all.

What Causes Fatigue?

Why does fatigue occur in people with MVPS/D? Unfortunately, the reason is not completely understood. There are theories, though. One theory relates to the functioning of the autonomic nervous system (ANS). It has been suggested that because of the imbalance of the ANS that accompanies MVPS/D, the blood vessels do not dilate or constrict properly (Phillips 1992). This can alter the proper blood flow to the entire body.

If the blood flow feeding and nourishing the large muscles of the body is restricted, there may be a build-up of a chemical called *lactic acid*. This lactic acid accumulates because the large muscles are not getting sufficient oxygen or nourishment, which may also contribute to a burning feeling in the muscles. Therefore, fatigue may be a result of a higher-than-normal production of lactic acid.

There are also some kinds of stress that cause or can contribute to fatigue. After all, living with any type of syndrome, day after day, can be emotionally draining, which in turn can lead to fatigue. Some of the types of emotional and physical stressors that contribute to fatigue are discussed below.

Depression

When you suffer from depression you may not feel like doing anything, going anywhere, or being with anyone, not even friends or family. When you are depressed, you may feel tired all the time. Conversely, being tired all the time can cause or increase depression. It's a self-perpetuating cycle that is sometimes difficult to escape.

It is important to distinguish true fatigue and poor exercise tolerance from the symptoms of depression. True fatigue and poor exercise tolerance may occur together with the symptoms of a clinical depression but they are a separate issue and must be addressed separately.

To tell the difference between the symptoms of clinical depression and the fatigue and inability to exercise symptomatic of MVPS/D, it can be useful to examine the symptoms of depression that specifically involve cognitive function. That is, if you are obsessing about how worthless you are, or how your life has no value, or if you are having persistent thoughts of suicide, and you are conscious of being depressed, then it is likely that you are experiencing clinical depression. If such is the case, you should seek treatment immediately. Major depression can be a major problem, but it is also one that has medical solutions.

Overextending Yourself

Some people describe their battles with fatigue this way:

Most of my fatigue comes from overdoing it. After all my years of living with MVPS/D, I still find it hard to pace myself. The fatigue is always there in varying degrees. Sometimes, it's difficult to know when I've reached my limit. I don't always listen to the signals of fatigue. The times when I feel good, I push myself too hard.

You may feel the same way. It's natural to want to keep up with your regular activities, but with MVPS/D this is not always possible. You are already going through life on overdrive because you have an excess of adrenaline and you are sensitive to adrenaline, so you're bound to feel more fatigued when you overextend yourself.

Hiding Your Symptoms From Others

You may not want others to know that you have MVPS/D. For that reason you may have developed the habit of pushing yourself extra hard to do the same things, at the same pace, that people without MVPS/D do. This usually results in hard "crashes," and having to "pay for it" later with extreme bouts of fatigue.

Analyze Your Fatigue

Learn to pace yourself so you won't become overtired. To do that, you need to know a lot about your body's reactions to everything. You need to analyze the way you live. At what time of day does your fatigue start? Is it worse at one time of day than at any other time? What adds to your fatigue? What helps to decrease it?

Are you consuming too much sugar? Remember, sugar will give you a momentary boost of energy at the cost of a terrible energy drain shortly after you ingest it. Are certain foods energizers? Are other foods energy depleters? Do mid-afternoon naps restore energy or do they sap it? How much sleep do you need? Eight hours? Nine hours? More? Everyone's body is different. Learn to listen to your body's signals telling you when it needs to rest.

Balance Rest and Activity

- **Learn your body's early signals that it is getting tired**. Take breaks during or between tasks, before you get too tired.

- **Pace yourself during the day**. Do a heavy task, then a light task, then another heavy task, and so on. Do the most difficult tasks when you're feeling your best, and you are at your highest energy level. If it takes a few days to accomplish a difficult task, so be it.

- **Know your priorities**. Focus on your top priorities while you have the energy. In this way, if fatigue sets in, it will be the less significant tasks that need to be delayed.

- **Don't try to do too much at one time**. Allow plenty of time to finish the things you start, so you won't feel rushed.

Make Your Work Easier

- **Plan ahead**. Look at all the tasks you do both at home and at work during a normal day and week. Eliminate the tasks that are not absolutely necessary. Delegate some of the others.

- **Create shortcuts**. Combine chores and errands, so you can get more done with less effort. For example, you can save time and energy by preparing several meals in advance. If you want to serve more complex meals, choose a day when you have more time and are feeling well.

- **Use labor-saving devices.** A microwave oven and/or a food processor can save you both time and energy. They are well worth the investment.

- **Organize work areas so you can get more done with less energy**. Arrange your desk or workspace with inexpensive storage bins. Keep all the equipment needed for a particular task together in one area. As a general rule, keep items you use most often closest to your work area and less-used items further away. If you are baking, store mixing bowls, sifter, measuring cups, and spoons in one place. If you are doing housework, keep cleaning supplies in several places: kitchen and bathroom, upstairs and downstairs.

Get Enough Sleep

Getting enough sleep when you have MVPS/D is often easier said than done. People with MVPS/D commonly report sleeping problems (Eiken 1991). The majority of the complaints seem to fall into the category of *insomnia*. Researchers define insomnia as inadequate or poor-quality sleep caused by one or several of the following problems:

- Difficulty falling asleep

- Waking up frequently at night and experiencing difficulty falling back asleep

- Waking up too early in the morning, and/or experiencing unrefreshing sleep (Wolfson 2001). This type of sleep pattern can be a significant contributing factor to increased daytime tiredness or fatigue.

Notice what inhibits your ability to sleep in your environment. Do low-level noises interfere? Does your partner frequently turn over in bed, or snore? Television noise from another room, or even the background noise from the street outside, can keep you from sleeping well. Low-level constant noise lessens the depth of sleep.

Consider using earplugs or sleeping in a separate bed in a quiet room. Sometimes a white noise machine can mask disturbing sounds. If you're sensitive to light, be sure your bedroom is very dark before you get into bed. If your mattress isn't comfortable, get a new one that is. You can make a too soft mattress firmer by putting a board beneath it. You can also make a hard mattress softer with an egg-crate foam pad. They are now available in any bedding store.

Good Sleep Hygiene

Good sleep hygiene involves changing your bedtime habits so that they're more conducive to sleep. The proper uses of beds are two: sleeping and lovemaking. Use your bed only for these two activities, not any others. Pay attention to how your naps affect you. Long periods of daytime resting and/or sleeping in your bed may change your ability to get to sleep at bedtime.

Give yourself a wind-down time before going to bed. During the pre-sleep hour, do activities that you know are going to make you sleepy, and do not do any mental and physical activities that stimulate you. Do not exercise or eat a large meal before going to sleep. On the other hand, taking a hot bath, or eating a light snack containing calcium before going to bed, may be sleep-inducing.

One essential ingredient for promoting restful sleep is setting and maintaining a daily routine of low-level mental and physical activities to help you distinguish daytime activities from those that are conducive to sleep at night. Create some rituals for getting ready for bed like lowering the blinds, turning off your telephone ringer, and so forth.

If you like to read before retiring, read something difficult and sleep-inducing, not a thriller—and read in an armchair, not your bed. Wear your pajamas or your bathrobe only at night, never during the day. Turn your phone off. If you set an alarm clock, do it at the same time every weekday night when you close the curtains or blinds. Rituals like these promote healthy sleep by preparing your mind to relax and let go of the day's activities.

Sleep Disorders and MVPS/D

A wide variety of sleep disorders exist that have the common symptoms of disrupted sleep, and subsequent excessive daytime sleepiness. Therefore, accurate diagnosis and treatment of your sleep problems often will require you to undergo all-night testing procedures that are conducted in a sleep disorders center.

A sleep disorders center evaluates people who have known or suspected sleep disorders. People with sleep disorders may present with complaints of insomnia, excessive daytime sleepiness, unusual movements or behaviors during sleep, nocturnal seizures, and disorders of the sleep/wake schedule.

To locate an accredited sleep disorder center in your state, you can go to www.aasmnet.org on the Internet. Once you have entered that home page address, you simply click on the state you live in, and any sleep disorder centers that are to be found in your state will be listed.

After a comprehensive evaluation and a consultation with a sleep specialist, you will be diagnosed and appropriate therapy will be determined. As part of the consultation and evaluation, a sleep study will be performed during a period of one or two nights. Hospitalization is not required, and overnight tests are usually completed by 7:00 A.M.

The testing procedure used is called *nocturnal polysomnography*. During the test, many different readings are taken from your body and are recorded during the night to determine the cause of your sleep disruption. These readings include EEG (brain waves), EMG (muscle activity), Rapid Eye Movement (REM sleep), and leg movement. In addition, your cardiac and respiratory activity are monitored and recorded throughout the night.

Note that people with MVPS/D are oftentimes very conscious or aware of the arousals and awakenings that occur during their sleep, and they can report the sleep-disrupting events quite descriptively (Eiken 1991).

One sleep-related event that appears to be significantly consistent among people with MVPS/D is the occurrence of an isolated respiratory event during the night. This event is characterized by a pause in breathing, associated with a sudden drop in the blood oxygen saturation level (Eiken 1991). This can result in an arousal or awakening that may also be accompanied by tachycardia and a sense of panic. This is known as a nocturnal panic attack.

It is also possible that hyperadrenergic stimulation may continue to occur during the night, and may be the cause of your disturbed sleep pattern. In other words, your adrenaline may keep "pumping" throughout the night.

Another type of sleep disorder that has been seen frequently in people with MVPS/D is *nocturnal myoclonus* (see chapter 3), or periodic limb movements during sleep (Eiken 1991). This disorder is characterized by frequent periodic twitching of the legs or arms during sleep, with associated arousals. As soon as you relax enough to fall asleep, your legs or arms begin to twitch and jerk. If the twitches are strong, or if you are a light sleeper, they disturb your sleep and wake you up. Obviously, if you have trouble falling asleep or if you wake up numerous times during the night due to these twitches you are likely to feel exhausted and sleepy during the day.

These sleep-related events (nocturnal panic attacks, hyperadrenergic stimulation, and nocturnal myoclonus) can result in disrupted sleep, and would certainly be consistent with a complaint of insomnia. These specific sleep disorders can be effectively diagnosed and treated at a sleep disorders center. In addition, there are some very simple preventive measures that can be followed that may be of benefit to people who suffer from the inability to fall asleep or to maintain sleep.

Treatment for Sleep Problems

First, the avoidance of all caffeine-containing food and drink is extremely important. Although the necessity for people with MVPS/D to avoid caffeine was discussed as extremely critical for other reasons (see chapter 7), ingesting caffeine also plays a significant role in disrupting sleep.

Exercising early in the morning and avoiding exercise or strenuous activities late in the day, can help you to sleep better. A good exercise program, which takes place at least four hours before bedtime, can be helpful for a good night's sleep. Avoiding alcohol prior to retiring for bed is also helpful. Alcohol may appear to promote sleep onset, but, in fact, it severely disrupts sleep during the course of the night.

Treatment for a sleep disorder may include a prescription for a device to aid breathing while sleeping, as well as some neuropsychiatric interventions, including biofeedback. In some people, a low dose of a benzodiazepine may be necessary to help restore normal sleep patterns. If indicated, referral to or consultations with other specialists might be recommended to aid in diagnosis and treatment.

If you have questions or concerns regarding your sleep, consult a physician at your local sleep disorders center. The polysomnography test is simple and noninvasive, and the potential for improving the quality of your life and your daytime functioning is quite dramatic.

Fatigue Breeds Fatigue

Lyn Frederickson, cofounder of The MVP Center in Birmingham, Alabama, when speaking about MVPS/D, always says, "Fatigue breeds fatigue." What she means is that, although you are more fatigued than people without MVPS/D, resting too much can actually increase your fatigue. Simply put, the less you do, the less you will feel like doing.

When symptoms occur and result in fatigue or other symptoms, you may have a tendency to do less and less. The old adage, "What you don't use, you lose," applies here. Your muscles need activity to remain strong. The cycle of fatigue must be broken by gently returning to physical activities and consistently striving to achieve a state of optimal conditioning.

Deconditioning results from prolonged inactivity. Therefore, there will be times when you simply will have to push yourself. You must learn to listen to all of your body's signals, so that you will know when to push yourself and when you truly have overdone it and need to rest. No one can tell you when you need to push and when you need to rest. You need to figure this out for yourself. But, in order to get "reconditioned," regular exercise is a must for you, not only to feel better, but to aid in easing many of your MVPS/D symptoms. Exercise is addressed in detail in chapter 11.

Emotional Support

In a healthy relationship, your partner will figure out a way to help you get the rest you need to recover your energy, so you will be able to complete some jobs without risking more fatigue than you can handle. You should try to do as much as you can without overextending yourself. Having an arrangement with your partner so that he or she will take over when you need to rest is a great idea, but if your partner doesn't have the time or energy to finish the task, let it go until the next day—or the next week, if that is the only time available. The measure of optimal support from your partner, both practical and emotional, is this: He or she gives you just the amount of support you want—not more and not less. The two of you will need to sit down and work out a plan that will allow you a mixture of support and independence. Too much support can present as much of a problem as too little support.

For your part, you do not want to encourage helplessness in yourself. Doing whatever you can to keep your independence and your household running smoothly will help you to maintain your self-respect, and will keep your partner from feeling resentment.

You know that you have had to make adjustments in your life to deal with MVPS/D. Stay aware that your partner also has had to make adjustments in his or her life to help you meet your needs. Consequently, there may be occasions when your partner becomes annoyed, or even angry, that you cannot do certain things. Clearly, for the good of your relationship as well as for your self-respect, it is essential to continue to do the things you can do. The more independent you can be, the happier you will be.

It is also important to find out what have been the most significant losses your partner has experienced. For example, companionship, child care, housework, sex, going out at night, and any number of other activities. Talk to your partner about how you can both change some of your priorities to make room to be together. Look for ways to nurture your life together.

In today's society, where many of you work more than forty hours a week, and run a household, and constantly shuttle children back and forth, you may think that reducing the fatigue you feel is an impossible task. This is simply not true. You *can* do it.

Although, initially, it may not be easy when you begin an exercise program and learn how to restructure your lifestyle, after only a few months of hard work and discipline, you will notice improvement. The longer you maintain your lifestyle modifications, especially your exercise program, the more significant your improvement will be.

If you don't think you have time to exercise, remember this—exercise reduces stress, increases energy, helps you sleep better, and improves vitality. Therefore, the time spent exercising pays benefits and interest by making the rest of your time more productive and less fatiguing.

CHAPTER 9

Panic Attacks

You understand, but fear flashes so fiercely you wilt before it.

—Claire Weekes

Joyce hopes to make it to her daughter's wedding this winter. This doesn't seem like a remarkable goal for a seemingly healthy person, but when sixty-year-old Joyce is anywhere near a crowd, she has a panic attack and wants to escape. In fact, Joyce has run out of wedding ceremonies in the past. That's because when she has a panic attack, she feels her heart beat as if it were bursting out of her chest. She also has hot flashes and chills, and experiences the fear of imminent death for the duration of the attack.

To hide her problem Joyce has made up many excuses. She told her family she was sick, so she wouldn't have to attend school plays and family gatherings. She told her sister that she was too busy to shop for Christmas presents, and her sister had to shop for her. But she is running out of excuses. As she said, "How many excuses can you give in a life?"

She went from doctor to doctor looking for an answer: Why did she fear crowds as much as she did? Finally, after suffering for nearly thirty years, Joyce was diagnosed as having panic disorder and as suffering from panic attacks.

Does this story sound familiar to you? Clearly, Joyce is not alone in her condition. Data compiled at the Mitral Valve Prolapse Center in Birmingham, Alabama, show that 70 percent of their mitral valve prolapse syndrome/dysautonomia (MVPS/D) patients have had panic attacks at some point in time (Watkins 1990).

Some of these patients have been virtually disabled because of the disorder, and they have become agoraphobic. This means that they have had to change their lifestyle completely. They stay at home where they feel safer and avoid going anywhere because of their fear of having a panic attack in a public place.

The Initial Panic Attack

Typically, a first panic attack seems to come "out of the blue." It can occur while you are engaged in an ordinary activity like walking to work or driving a car. You can be struck suddenly by a barrage of frightening and uncomfortable symptoms. These symptoms often can include feeling terror, a sense of unreality, the fear of losing control, and the usual MVPS/D symptoms including heart palpitations and tachycardia. This barrage of symptoms usually lasts several seconds, but it can continue for several minutes. Over the course of about an hour the symptoms gradually fade.

People with MVPS/D who have experienced panic attacks attest to feeling intense physical discomfort and to fearing that they have been stricken with some terrible, life-threatening disease or are "going mad." They often seek help at hospital emergency rooms.

When in the middle of a panic attack, many people with MVPS/D believe that the heart attack that they have always feared is finally happening. After spending some time in an emergency room undergoing various physical examinations, they are usually told their heart is fine and that they've had a panic attack.

Initial panic attacks also can occur when you are experiencing a great deal of stress, from an overload of work, for example, or from the loss of a family member or close friend. Panic attacks can follow surgery, a serious accident, illness, or childbirth. Excessive consumption of caffeine or the use of cocaine and other stimulant drugs can set off a panic attack. So can the use of medicines, such as the stimulants used for treating asthma. This is especially true for people with MVPS/D because of their sensitivity to adrenaline. When stimulants are used, the body produces more adrenaline.

Nevertheless, despite these many different kinds of triggers, a panic attack usually takes you completely by surprise. This unpredictability is one reason the attacks are so devastating. Those who do not have MVPS/D and who have never had a panic attack sometimes assume that the panic felt in a panic attack is just a matter of feeling intensely nervous or anxious, the sort of feelings with which everyone is familiar.

In fact, even though you may not show any outward signs of terror during a panic attack, the feelings you experience are so overwhelming and terrifying that you really believe you are going to die,

lose your mind, or be totally humiliated. These disastrous consequences don't occur, but when you are having a panic attack, they
seem quite likely.

Some people who have one panic attack, or an occasional
attack, never develop a problem serious enough for it to greatly
affect their lives. For others, however, the panic attacks continue and
cause much grief and suffering.

Symptoms of a Panic Attack

During a panic attack, some or all of the following symptoms
occur:

- Terror—the sense that something unimaginably horrible is
  about to happen and you are powerless to prevent it

- Racing or pounding heartbeat

- Chest pains

- Dizziness, lightheadedness, nausea

- Difficulty breathing

- Tingling or numbness in the hands

- Flushes or chills

- Sense of unreality

- Fear of losing control, going crazy, or doing something
  embarrassing

- Fear of dying

Strategies for Coping with Panic Attacks

1. Remember that this is not a sign of weakness or personal
   failure.

2. Remember that although your feelings and symptoms are
   very frightening, they are not dangerous or harmful.

3. Do not fight your feelings or try to wish them away. The
   more you are willing to face them, the less intense they will
   become.

4. Stay in the present. Notice what is really happening to you
   as opposed to what you think might happen.

5. When the fear comes, expect and accept it. Wait and give it time to pass without running away from it.

6. Be proud of yourself for your progress thus far, and think about how good you will feel when you succeed this time.

Panic Disorder

In the condition called *panic disorder*, panic attacks recur and you develop an intense apprehension of having another attack. This particular fear, which is called *anticipatory anxiety* or *fear of fear*, can be present most of the time and thus seriously interfere with your life, even when a panic attack is not in progress. In addition, you may develop phobias about situations where a panic attack has occurred. For example, if you have had a panic attack while driving, you may be afraid to get behind the wheel again, even to drive to the grocery store.

If you develop such panic-induced phobias, you will tend to avoid the situations that you fear will trigger a panic attack and, as a result, your life may become increasingly limited. Your work may suffer because you can't travel or get to work on time. Relationships may be strained or marred by conflict as panic attacks, or the fear of them, rule over you and those close to you.

Your sleep may be disturbed because of panic attacks that take place at night, causing you to awaken in a state of terror. This experience is so harrowing that some people who have nocturnal panic attacks become afraid to go to sleep and suffer from exhaustion. Furthermore, even if you don't have nocturnal panic attacks, your sleep may be disturbed because of chronic, panic-related anxiety. Obviously, this means more trouble for people with MVPS/D who already suffer from fatigue.

Many people with panic disorder remain intensely concerned about their symptoms even after a visit to a physician yields no indication of a life-threatening condition. These people may visit a succession of doctors seeking medical treatment for what they believe is heart disease or a respiratory problem. To compound the problem, people who have panic disorder, and are aware that they have structural MVP, usually believe that they have developed some type of heart disease.

Panic disorder tends to distort one's perceptions. This means that those with MVPS/D must realize that if they were not suffering from panic disorder, the physical problems associated with MVPS/D would seem far less profound. In other words, when they developed symptoms like headaches or stomach pains, they wouldn't blow them out of proportion and convince themselves they had brain tumors, or ulcers, or cancer.

Since people with MVPS/D also respond to stimuli more intensely than other people do (see chapter 2), all objectivity is lost, and they begin to dwell on the first negative thought that "pops" into their brain at any given moment.

The search for medical help may continue for a long time, because physicians who see these patients often fail to diagnose panic disorder. And when doctors do recognize the condition, they sometimes explain it in terms that suggest it is of no importance or not treatable.

For example, many people with MVPS/D have had a doctor say to them, "There's nothing to worry about. You're just having a panic attack," or "It's just nerves." Although meant to be reassuring, such words can be very disturbing to the worried person whose symptoms keep recurring. That person needs to know that panic disorder is a recognized disorder and that it can be treated effectively.

Agoraphobia

If left untreated, panic disorder may progress to a more advanced stage, one in which you become afraid of being in any place or situation where, in the event of a panic attack, escape might be difficult for you or no help would be available. This condition is called agoraphobia. It affects about a third of all people who have panic disorder (National Institute of Mental Health 1995).

Typically, people with agoraphobia fear being in crowds, standing in line, entering shopping malls, and riding in cars or public transportation. Often, agoraphobics restrict themselves to a "safety zone" that may include only their home or the immediate neighborhood. Any movement beyond the edges of this zone creates mounting anxiety.

Sometimes a person with agoraphobia is unable to leave home alone, but can travel if accompanied by a particular family member or friend. Even when they restrict themselves to "safe" situations, most people with agoraphobia continue to have panic attacks at least a few times a month (National Institute of Mental Health 1995).

People with agoraphobia can be seriously disabled by their condition. Some are unable to work, and they may need to rely heavily on other family members, who must do the shopping and run all the household errands, as well as accompany the affected person on rare excursions outside the "safety zone." Thus, the person with agoraphobia typically leads a life of extreme dependency as well as one of great discomfort.

Treatment for Panic Disorder

Treatment can bring significant relief to 70 to 90 percent of people with panic disorder, and early treatment can help to prevent the disease from progressing to its later stages where agoraphobia develops (National Institute of Mental Health 1995).

Before undergoing any treatment for panic disorder, you should first have a thorough medical examination to rule out any other possible causes of the distressing symptoms. This is essential because other conditions, such as excessive levels of thyroid hormone, certain types of epilepsy, or cardiac arrhythmias can cause symptoms resembling those of panic disorder, but they require very different forms of treatment.

Cognitive-Behavioral Therapy

Cognitive-behavioral therapy is a combination of *cognitive therapy*, which can modify or eliminate the thought patterns that contribute to your symptoms, and *behavioral therapy*, which aims at helping you to change your behavior, i.e., your habitual patterns.

The "cognitive model" for panic attacks maintains that people with panic disorder often have serious distortions in their thinking, of which they may be unaware, and that these distortions may give rise to a cycle of fear (National Institute of Mental Health 1995). The cycle is believed to operate in the following way:

- First the individual with panic disorder feels a potentially worrisome sensation, such as an increasing heart rate, tightened chest muscles, or a queasy stomach.

- Second, the person responds to the sensation by becoming anxious. This initial anxiety triggers still more unpleasant sensations, which in turn heighten the anxiety, giving rise to catastrophic thoughts. The person thinks "I am having a heart attack" or "I am going insane," or some similar thought.

- As the cycle continues, a full-blown panic attack results. The whole cycle might take only a few seconds to complete itself, and the person may not be aware of the initial sensations or thoughts.

Proponents of this theory point out that with the help of a skilled therapist, you can learn to recognize your earliest thoughts and feelings in this sequence, and thus modify your responses to them. You are taught that typical thoughts like, "This terrible feeling is getting worse!" or "I'm going to have a panic attack or a heart attack" can be replaced with substitutes like, "This is only uneasiness—it will pass" that help to reduce anxiety and ward off a panic attack. By modifying your thought patterns in this way, you gain more control over the problem.

The "behavioral" portion of cognitive-behavioral therapy may involve systematic training in relaxation techniques. By learning to relax, you may acquire the ability to reduce the generalized anxiety and stress that often set the stage for panic attacks.

Frequently, breathing exercises are also included in the behavioral aspect of cognitive-behavioral therapy. You learn to control your breathing and to avoid hyperventilation, which is a pattern of rapid, shallow breathing that can trigger or exacerbate some panic attacks.

"*In vivo*" or *real-life* exposure is another important aspect of behavioral therapy. For this work, you and your therapist determine whether you have been avoiding particular places and situations, and which patterns of avoidance are causing you problems. You both agree to work on the avoidance behaviors that seriously interfere with your life. For example, fear of driving may be of paramount importance for you, while the inability to go to the grocery store may be the issue of most importance for another person.

Exposure therapy requires the patient to "expose" himself or herself to the feared situation several or many times until the situation no longer has the power to arouse fear. Some cognitive-behavioral therapists will come to your home to conduct the initial sessions.

More often, cognitive-behavioral therapists take their patients on excursions to shopping malls, movies, and other public places that their patients have been avoiding. Or they may accompany those who are trying to overcome fear of driving in the car. They sit in the passenger seat and say calming and soothing words while the patient drives along city streets or freeways.

The patient approaches a fearful situation gradually, always trying to stay in the feared situation—the exposure—in spite of rising levels of anxiety. At each exposure, the patient tries to stay in the feared situation feeling whatever feelings come up and not fleeing.

In this way the patient sees that, as frightening as the feelings are, they are not dangerous, and they do pass. Patients find that with this step-by-step approach, aided by encouragement and skilled advice from the therapist, they can master their fears gradually and go places and do things that previously were not available to them.

Treatment with Medication

In this treatment approach, which is also called *pharmaco-therapy*, a prescription medication is used to prevent panic attacks, or to reduce their frequency and severity, and to decrease the associated anticipatory anxiety. When you find that your panic attacks are less frequent and less severe, you will be able to venture into situations that were previously off-limits to you. In this way, you can benefit from exposing yourself to feared situations as well as from the medication.

The three groups of medications most commonly used for panic disorder are the selective serotonin reuptake inhibitors (SSRIs), tricyclic antidepressants, and benzodiazepines. Determination of which drug to use is based on considerations of safety, efficacy, and your personal needs and preferences. Some information about each of these classes of drugs follows.

SSRIs

Selective serotonin reuptake inhibitors (SSRIs) such as Prozac, Zoloft, and Paxil are becoming the treatment of choice for panic. They help to control the symptoms of anxiety and panic by regulating the balance of serotonin in the brain (Hedaya 2000). The SSRIs are more easily tolerated than the older tricyclic antidepressants, which means that people are more likely to stay on them long enough to see good results. And, unlike the benzodiazepines, SSRIs have no potential for abuse and don't produce dependence. People generally start with very low doses of SSRIs to avoid overstimulation and sleep disturbances. The dosage can be increased over several weeks.

Tricyclic Antidepressants

The tricyclic antidepressants were the first medications demonstrated to have a beneficial effect against panic disorder (Hedaya 2000). Imipramine is the tricyclic most commonly used for panic disorder.

When imipramine is prescribed, you usually start with small daily doses that are increased every few days until an effective dosage is reached. This slow introduction of imipramine helps to minimize the side effects such as dry mouth, constipation, and blurred vision that are frequently present. People with panic disorder who are inclined to be hypervigilant about physical sensations, such as people with MVPS/D, often find these side effects disturbing at the outset. These side effects usually fade away after you have been on the medication a few weeks.

It usually takes several weeks for imipramine to have a beneficial effect on panic disorder. Most people treated with imipramine will be panic-free within a few weeks or months (National Institute of Mental Health 1995). Treatment generally lasts from six to twelve months. Treatment for a shorter period of time is possible, but there is substantial risk that when the imipramine is stopped, the panic attacks will recur. Extending the period of treatment to six months to indefinitely may reduce this risk of a relapse. When the treatment period is complete, the dosage of imipramine is tapered down over a period of several weeks.

Benzodiazepines

The benzodiazepines are a class of medications that effectively reduce anxiety. Alprazolam, clonazepam, and lorazepam are medications that belong to this class. They take effect rapidly and are usually well tolerated by the majority of people who use them. However, some people, especially those who have had problems with alcohol or drug dependency, may become dependent on benzodiazepines.

Generally, the physician prescribing one of these drugs starts the patient on a low dose and gradually raises it until the panic attacks cease. This procedure minimizes side effects. Treatment with benzodiazepines is usually continued for six months to a year. One drawback to this treatment is that you may experience withdrawal symptoms such as malaise, weakness, and other such unpleasant effects when the treatment is discontinued. Reducing the dose gradually generally minimizes these problems. There may also be a recurrence of panic attacks after the medication is withdrawn.

As in the case of the SSRIs and imipramine, treatment with benzodiazepines generally lasts six months to a year, but longer treatment may be needed depending on the person's response. At the conclusion of the treatment period, the medication is gradually tapered off.

When Panic Recurs

Panic disorder can be a chronic illness with many recoveries and many relapses. For many, it gets better at some times and worse at others. If a person receives treatment, and appears to have overcome the problem, it can still worsen later for no apparent reason. These recurrences should not cause anyone to despair or consider himself or herself a "treatment failure." Recurrences can be treated just as effectively as an initial panic attack.

In fact, the skills that a person can learn from dealing with an initial episode of terror can be helpful in coping with any setbacks. Many people who have overcome panic disorder one or more times have found that they are now much better able to deal with the problem. Even though it may not be fully cured, panic no longer dominates their lives, or the lives of those around them.

Referrals to Professional Help

The people and places that will make a referral or provide diagnostic and treatment services to someone with the symptoms described in this chapter are listed below. Also check the Yellow Pages under "mental health," "anxiety," "suicide prevention," "hospitals," "physicians," "psychiatrists," "psychologists," or "social workers" for addresses and phone numbers.

- Family doctors

- Mental health specialists, such as psychiatrists, psychologists, social workers, or mental health counselors

- Health maintenance organizations

- Community mental health centers

- Hospital psychiatry departments and outpatient clinics

- Family service/social agencies

- Employee assistance programs

- Local medical, psychiatric, or psychological societies

Finding Help for Panic Disorder

Often the person with panic disorder must strenuously search to find a doctor who is familiar with the most effective treatments for the condition. The Anxiety Disorders Association of America (see Resources) can provide a list of professionals in your area who specialize in the treatment of panic disorder and other anxiety disorders.

Support Groups

Self-help and support groups are the least expensive approach to managing panic disorder and have proved helpful to some people. In these groups, a small number of people meet weekly and share their experiences, encouraging each other to venture into feared situations to learn to cope effectively with panic attacks.

Group members are in charge of the sessions. Often family members are invited to attend these group meetings, and at times, a physician or other panic disorder expert may be brought in to share insights and information with group members. Information on self-help groups in specific areas of the country can be obtained from the Anxiety Disorders Association of America.

What to Do if a Family Member Has an Anxiety Disorder

- Don't make assumptions about what the affected person needs; ask the person.

- Be predictable; don't surprise the person.

- Let the person with the disorder set the pace for recovery.

- Find something positive in every experience. If the affected person is able to go only part of the way to a particular goal, such as going to a movie or party, consider that the effort alone is an achievement, rather than a failure.

- Don't enable avoidance: Negotiate with the person to take one step forward when he or she wants to avoid something.

- Don't panic when the person with the disorder panics.

- Be patient and accepting, but don't settle for the affected person being permanently disabled.

- Don't say, "Relax. Calm down. Don't be anxious. Let's see if you can do this" (i.e., don't set up a test for the affected person). Comments like, "You can fight this, What should we do next, Don't be ridiculous, You *have* to stay, and Don't be a coward," all do more harm than good.

Goals for the Person with Panic Disorder

Your goal should be to control your panic attacks. If cognitive therapy, breathing techniques, and exposure therapy do not bring the kind of relief you want, you have the option of taking medication. In fact, after you have been on medication for a while it is often much easier to implement the lifestyle modifications needed to get your nervous system back into balance.

Because there is a biological component to panic (Phillips 1992), it may be necessary to treat panic with medications. These medications block whatever is biochemically contributing to the onset or to the exacerbation of your panic attacks.

Don't feel as if you are demonstrating a weak character if you decide to take medication or consult with a therapist. You should feel strong in the knowledge that you are taking an active role in regaining control over your life and in controlling your MVPS/D.

CHAPTER 10

Medications

Medicine is the science of uncertainty, and the art of probability.

—E. Mumford

If you have tried all of the lifestyle modifications that have been suggested for treating your mitral valve prolapse syndrome/ dysautonomia (MVPS/D) and you are still symptomatic, you are likely to be a good candidate for medication. This is especially true if you are suffering from anxiety, panic disorder, and/or depression. Remember, this does not mean that somehow you are weak; nor does it mean that you will have to take medications for the rest of your life.

There are different degrees of MVPS/D. You may know someone with MVPS/D who has few, if any, problems, while your symptoms may be totally disabling. Therefore, you may require medication while that person may be able to control his or her MVPS/D simply by exercising and changing his or her diet.

Unfortunately, there is still a stigma attached to taking psychiatric medications. Many people still say, "I don't want to have to rely on medication." But taking medication for MVPS/D, such as an SSRI, may help to balance the neurotransmitters and other chemicals in your brain, much in the same way that people with diabetes take insulin to normalize the sugar levels in their blood. We are lucky to be living in a time when there are so many medications available.

Pharmaceuticals

The following medications may be prescribed for the treatment of MVPS/D. Included in these discussions are some of the most common side effects that each type of medication may have.

Beta-Blockers

Beta-blockers can be very effective for alleviating some of the most disturbing symptoms of MVPS/D, namely tachycardia and palpitations. They may also lessen anxiety, chest pain, and migraine headaches.

- Tenormin
- Corgard
- Inderal
- Lopressor
- Kerlone
- Zebeta
- Toprol

Because people with MVPS/D tend to need only a low dose of a beta-blocker, side effects are limited. Beta-blockers may not be suitable for people who suffer from asthma, hay fever, emphysema, or chronic bronchitis.

Side Effects of Beta-Blockers

The common side effects experienced by those who take beta-blockers include the following: slow pulse, drowsiness, fatigue, weakness, dizziness, and nightmares.

Benzodiazepines

Benzodiazepines belong to the class of medicines called central nervous system depressants. They are used to relieve anxiety and sometimes insomnia. One of the reasons they are used for panic disorder is because they are fast-acting.

- Klonopin
- Librax

- Librium

- Xanax

- Ativan

- Valium

Benzodiazepines have few side effects when taken as directed. However, they can be addictive and should not be stopped abruptly if taken for a long period of time. Benzodiazepines are not appropriate for people with alcohol or other substance abuse problems.

Side Effects of Benzodiazepines

The common side effects experienced by those who take benzodiazepines include the following: clumsiness or unsteadiness, dizziness or light-headedness, drowsiness, and slurred speech.

Anti-Anxiety Agent: BuSpar

BuSpar is a medication used primarily for relief of mild to moderate anxiety and nervous tension. It is useful in treating the elderly and people with substance abuse problems. Alcohol does not interact in a dangerous manner with BuSpar. In fact, it may be useful in reducing alcohol craving. BuSpar is sometimes used in addition to an SSRI to combat the SSRI's side effect of decreased libido. It is not addictive, but unlike the benzodiazepines it may take several weeks to notice results.

Side Effects of BuSpar

The common side effects of BuSpar include the following: chest pain, excitability, headaches, dream disturbances (i.e., nightmares), dizziness, light-headedness, and ringing in the ears.

Antidepressants

Although antidepressants are best known for treating depression they are also commonly used for treating other conditions such as panic attacks, generalized anxiety disorder (GAD), severe premenstrual syndrome (PMS), fibromyalgia, irritable bowel syndrome (IBS), obsessive-compulsive disorder (OCD), restless leg syndrome, migraines, and attention deficit disorder (ADD).

The biochemical reality is that all classes of medication that treat depression (SSRIs, tricyclic antidepressants, and atypical antidepressants) have some effect on norepinephrine and serotonin, as well as on other neurotransmitters in the brain. However, the various medications affect the different neurotransmitters in varying degrees.

Tricyclic Antidepressants

Tricyclic antidepressants (TCAs) were developed in the 1950s and 1960s to treat depression. They work mainly by increasing the level of norepinephrine in the brain's synapses. They also affect serotonin levels. Tricyclic antidepressants are safe and are generally well-tolerated. However, if taken in an overdose, TCAs can cause life-threatening heart rhythm disturbances.

- Anafranil

- Elavil

- Pamelor

- Sinequan

- Imipramine

Side Effects of TCAs

There are a number of possible side effects with tricyclic antidepressants, but they vary depending on the medication. Because of this variation in side effects one TCA may be highly desirable for one person and contraindicated for another. Many side effects may disappear quickly, while others will remain for the duration of the treatment. It usually takes two to five weeks to notice improvement.

The common side effects of the TCAs include the following: dry mouth, constipation, dizziness, blurred vision, and muscle twitches.

Atypical Antidepressants

Atypical antidepressants are so named because they work in a variety of ways. Thus, atypical antidepressants are not TCAs or SSRIs, but they work like them. They increase the level of certain neurochemicals in the brain's synapses.

Wellbutrin is sometimes used in addition to an SSRI to combat the SSRI's side effect of a decreased libido. Wellbutrin, also known as Zyban, can also be used to combat an addiction to cigarettes.

If you are prescribed Serzone or Effexor make sure your physician knows about any other medications you are taking. Serzone can be especially dangerous when combined with Xanax and BuSpar. All of the atypical antidepressants need to be taken for two to five weeks before you see an improvement in the condition for which you are taking the medication.

- Effexor

- Wellbutrin

- Serzone

- Desyrel

Side Effects of Atypical Antidepressants

Common side effects of atypical antidepressants include the following: sleep disturbances, dry mouth, agitation, anxiety, nervousness, chest pain, and dizziness.

Selective Serotonin Reuptake Inhibitors

Selective serotonin reuptake inhibitors (SSRIs) affect serotonin, one of the most important neurotransmitters in the brain. Serotonin plays a role in governing the emotions and in psychological disturbances. The SSRIs have fewer side effects than tricyclic antidepressants. The side effects caused by SSRIs generally disappear within the first month of use. It will take two to five weeks to notice an improvement.

- Prozac

- Paxil

- Zoloft

- Celexa

- Luvox

Side Effects of the SSRIs

Common side effects of the SSRIs include the following: nausea, diarrhea, agitation, insomnia, headaches, and decreased libido.

MVPS/D and Over-the-Counter (OTC) Medications

The majority of people with MVPS/D learn quickly that they are unusually sensitive to most medications and, as a result, they become reluctant to take medications that have been prescribed for them. However, there are times when you have a headache, the flu, or a cold, for example, in which an over-the-counter drug can be very effective. The secret is to use a drug that is not only effective but also does not aggravate the symptoms of MVPS/D. Note that there are some over-the-counter medications that can increase your heart rate or worsen your chest pain.

Generally, it is safer to select single-ingredient agents rather than ones that have several components. For example, it is better to take an aspirin and a plain decongestant for a cold or sinus congestion than one of the many cold preparations on the market that contains multiple ingredients, especially those containing caffeine and ephedrine, such as pseudoephedrine.

Your pharmacist can be a good resource for you, so if you're unsure of the ingredients in an over-the-counter medication, ask her or him whether it is safe for someone with MVP to take that medication. Note that if all OTC cold medications cause you to become symptomatic, you should ask your physician for a prescription cold medication that will be safe for you.

Be aware of the over-the-counter drugs that contain large amounts of caffeine. Excedrin contains 65 milligrams of caffeine. Anacin and Midol contain 32 milligrams. NoDoz contains 100 milligrams, and Vivarin contains 200 milligrams of caffeine. Taking any one of these may exacerbate your MVPS/D symptoms.

Diet Pills

As a general rule, stay away from diet pills. This includes natural products that are advertised as being fat burners. The problem with them is the frequency and severity of their side effects. They may cause anxiety, depression, insomnia, irritability, delusions, elevated blood pressure, rapid heart rate, palpitations, headaches, and gastrointestinal disturbances.

Herbal Remedies

The popularity of natural herbal remedies has increased enormously in the last few years. That may be due to the common belief that natural products are always healthy and safe to consume. However, little is known about the toxicity and pharmacological interactions of many of these substances. Remember, tobacco and arsenic are also natural products. Always consult your physician before using any herbal product.

The following herbal ingredients should be avoided unless your physician specifically states that it would be safe for you to take them.

- Mahaung: This contains ephedrine and pseudoephedrine, which naturally increase blood pressure and heart rate and stimulate metabolism. Mahaung can be potentially life-threatening.

- Kola nut: This contains caffeine.

- Guarana: This contains caffeine.

- Passion flower: This can cause depression, nervousness, and stimulation of the nervous system.

- Ginseng: This has a diuretic effect; it may also cause insomnia and arrhythmias, and worsen hypertension.

- Licorice: This has a diuretic effect.

- Ginkgo biloba: This may lower blood pressure.

- St. John's Wort: This can be toxic when used in combination with antidepressants.

- Yohimbine: This can cause panic attacks, anxiety, palpitations, and nervousness, especially when combined with antidepressants.

MVPS/D and Medications

Miscellaneous medications may be prescribed to treat various MVPS/D symptoms including irritable bowel syndrome (IBS), migraines, esophageal reflux, insomnia, PMS, and hypotension. Everyone is unique biochemically. Therefore, the occurrence of side effects or the lack of a satisfactory result with one type of medication does not mean that another medication in the same class will not be beneficial.

A lot of people with MVPS/D become frustrated taking prescribed medications because of their side effects. Unfortunately, prescribing the proper medication and dosage is not an exact science. Therefore, you and your doctor must work together and be persistent in determining which medication is best for you. You should contact your physician as soon as you experience a side effect and then follow his or her instructions.

Many people simply stop taking their medication without even informing their doctor of the side effects it is causing. This can be dangerous because some medications cannot be stopped "cold turkey." You may need to gradually lower the dosage to be weaned from them. Also, sometimes you must take the medication for a certain duration of time before it becomes effective.

As frustrating as side effects can be, they do go away with certain medications if you take them for a long enough period of time. Nevertheless, if a side effect is particularly troublesome, your doctor may prescribe a different medication for you. It is not easy to change medications two or three different times, but it is not unusual before the right medication for you is prescribed at the right dosage.

If you and your physician are willing to work together diligently to find the proper medication to treat your MVPS/D, it will be worth all of the time and effort it takes. The difference in your life that can be made by taking the most appropriate and effective medication for yourself is remarkable.

Some people with MVPS/D say, "I'm too young to be on medication. I look perfectly normal and healthy. Why should I take medication?" To this question, we respond by asking you, "Would you say the same thing to a diabetic?" An imbalance in the nervous system and in the brain is just as much of a physical problem as diabetes is. The main difference is that many medications for MVPS/D must be prescribed by a psychiatrist.

Hopefully, sometime in the near future our society will erase the stigma of going to psychiatrists and taking psychiatric medication. Until that time comes, it remains deeply unfortunate that some people feel a need to hide their disorder or the medications they take to deal with that disorder because of the stigma. Seeking psychiatric drugs for particular disorders is no more and no less sensible than seeking medical help for diabetes or for heart trouble.

CHAPTER 11

Modifying Your Lifestyle

There is no failure except in no longer trying.
—Elbert Hubbard

You've now learned something about the complexities of mitral valve prolapse syndrome/dysautonomia (MVPS/D) and its numerous symptoms. It is a lot of material to digest. Try not to let it overwhelm you. Even though you may need to make many lifestyle modifications, there is no need to change everything overnight. Take it slowly, one day at a time. If you have panic attacks, panic disorder, and/or depression, you will probably want to get that condition under control first. It is much easier to implement lifestyle modifications like starting an exercise program and changing your diet if you first feel emotionally fit. Later, as you begin to notice improvements in your MVPS/D symptoms, you can then slowly add other changes to your life.

The Role of Exercise

The importance of exercise in treating MVPS/D cannot be overemphasized. Aerobic exercise is one of the key methods for getting your nervous system back in balance. Exercising can alleviate fatigue, anxiety, and depression, and help you to get a better night's sleep (Luketic and Watkins 2000).

We all know we should exercise to be healthy, and we all know that it is an important component in the preventive management of health problems, especially for managing many of the symptoms of MVPS/D. So, if it's so good for you, why isn't everyone exercising?

There are several answers to that question. Some people say they can't find the time. But nearly everyone can carve half an hour out of every day. Really motivated people who are short of time run in place while watching the morning news on TV. The trick is in becoming motivated.

Some people find that following a regular exercise routine is boring and difficult to maintain. If exercise seems like "work," then you probably won't stick with it. The key to staying motivated is to find something you like to do—or several somethings.

You may not like to run, either in place, or in marathons, but how about dancing? Many women get aerobic exercise by dancing—either alone in their home or with a partner on a dance floor. Be creative. Find a way to move aerobically that gives you pleasure and you will become motivated to exercise regularly.

Realizing some of the benefits of exercise doesn't have to mean embarking on an intense training program. You should participate in any activity that is continuous, nonstop, and moderately strenuous (walking, swimming, aerobics classes, dancing) three to five times a week for thirty to forty-five minutes (Luketic and Watkins 2000). That is a general guideline.

If you are just starting to exercise, thirty minutes might be too much for you. Instead, you can progress to this level gradually by starting with five to ten minute sessions to build endurance and then work up to twenty to thirty minutes. Participate in activities that match your ability and current fitness level. Of course you should check your health with your physician before beginning any exercise program.

What Is Perceived Exertion?

All around the country, posted on the walls of health clubs alongside the treadmills, stationary bikes, and step machines, you will often see a scale numbered from 6 to 20. This is called an RPE Scale, which stands for "Rate of Perceived Exertion." It is a psychophysiological scale, meaning that the scale uses both your mind and body to rate your perception of your efforts.

This scale is designed to help you estimate the intensity level of your exercise (that is, how your exercise or activity "feels" while you are performing it). For example, sitting in a chair would be perceived to be a "very, very light" activity, graded around 6 or 7 on the Perceived Exertion Scale.

Getting up and walking easily across the room might be estimated as "very light," and it would be around 8 or 9 on the scale. Walking at a moderate pace is "fairly light" and it would receive a rating of around 10 or 11. Picking up your pace to a brisk walk might be perceived as "somewhat hard" and would be graded at about 13. Walking as fast as possible might feel like a 14, and if it causes breathlessness, a 15. It is recommended that you should not exercise to this level of "breathlessness" (above level 14).

When exercising, you should monitor your intensity by using a perceived exertion scale to make sure that you're not working too hard. Using this scale is a good way for people with MVPS/D to monitor their workouts. For example, if you have tachycardia, you will not be able to gauge your intensity level simply by taking your pulse, because your pulse may *always* be rapid, during exercise and while at rest.

Alternatively, you may be taking a type of medication that doesn't allow your pulse to fluctuate very much no matter what you do. In both of these cases you would not be able to get a "true" reading of your intensity level unless you used a perceived exertion scale.

Therefore, pace your activity or exercise within this training zone of "feeling" as if you were exerting yourself somewhere between "fairly light" and a little more than "somewhat hard," (11–14) but not to the point of being short of breath. You should be able to talk to a friend while you exercise.

Perceived Exertion Scale

The level of perceived exertion is often measured with a 15-category scale that was developed by Swedish psychologist Gunnar Borg (Utter, Kang, and Robertson 2001). The Borg scale is shown below:

6	Very, very light
7	Very, very light
8	Very light
9	Very light
10	Very light
11	Fairly light
12	Fairly light
13	Somewhat hard
14	Somewhat hard
15	Hard

16   Hard

17   Very hard

18   Very hard

19   Very, very hard

20   Very, very hard

Exercising should be enjoyable, stimulating, and invigorating so that you look forward to your regular activity. Exercising too hard causes people to drop out of exercising.

How Can I Make Myself Exercise When I'm So Fatigued All The Time?

If you haven't been active for a while, you should see your doctor before starting an exercise program. You should start out slowly. For example, you could first try just walking for a few minutes each day. Start out slowly with small goals, like just walking around the block the first day of your new program. Then, on the second day, add another block. On the third day, another. . . .

In the beginning, you may find that you're more fatigued after your walk than you were before you went outside. And you may have to force yourself to take a walk the next day because you would much rather take a nap. But if you can stick with it for several weeks, you'll discover that you have more energy. You'll see that, no matter how tired you get, each day you walk (or work out) you will gain in strength and stamina.

How Can Exercising Give Me More Energy?

One reason for the increase you will experience in your energy level is that aerobic exercise makes your heart stronger and causes it to work more efficiently. A fit cardiovascular system delivers more oxygen per minute during physical exertion and at rest than an unfit system (Sullivan 2001). Also, stronger muscles give you the endurance to get through the day with energy to spare. Furthermore, exercise can improve the quality of your sleep, so you will feel better rested, even after spending the same amount of time in bed.

If My Muscles Are Screaming and I'm Gasping for Breath in the First Few Minutes, Should I Keep Going?

The answer is an emphatic "no." You should slow down and catch your breath. Once you feel more comfortable you can start slowly building up your pace. Your muscles may hurt at first because they're producing lactic acid (see chapter 8).

If you've been spending a lot of time on the couch, your lungs aren't used to having to boost their oxygen intake at a moment's notice. But once you've built up a little endurance, your breathing should catch up with your efforts, giving your muscles the oxygen they need. The better shape you're in, the sooner you'll reach this state.

How Can I Make Myself Exercise When I'm So Depressed?

If you are suffering from depression, talk to your doctor first about psychotherapy or medication, or both. After you start to feel a little better, you might look for a structured group exercise program built around activities that you've enjoyed doing in the past or that you think you might enjoy now.

Joining a walking group is often a good option because you can be at any fitness level and you don't need any training or special equipment. You may need to keep at it for several weeks before noticing an improvement in your mood, but try to make it a habit you don't want to give up. Remember, exercise is not a substitute for other kinds of treatment for depression, but it's a good complementary activity to add to your treatment regimen.

Endorphins

The theory goes that when you exercise intensely the stress on your body prompts your brain to release substances called endorphins into your bloodstream. These endorphins attach themselves onto nerve receptors all over your body, blocking pain signals. They may cause you to feel euphoric and simultaneously relaxed and energized, even hours after you've stopped exercising.

A leisurely walk around the block probably won't release endorphins. The exercise has to be more intense than that, but any kind of regular activity will give you more energy on a day-to-day basis. You don't have to become addicted to endorphins to benefit.

Patience Is a Virtue

Be patient. It has probably taken you quite a long time to become deconditioned. It will also take a while to get back in shape. It won't happen overnight, but gradually you will begin to feel much better.

Stress

Stress is an unavoidable part of our existence. Feeling it is the body's natural reaction to an experience or a challenge. The body responds to stress in mental, physical, chemical, and emotional ways. Stress may be constructive and motivational or destructive and dangerous to health. Stress alone is not the problem. How stress affects you depends largely on how you react to what happens to you.

One major problem caused by our multiple reactions to stress is that often these reactions are no longer appropriate to the triggering events. When we experience danger, a bodily reaction is triggered called the "fight or flight response." This is our body's automatic, innate response that prepares us to fight or flee from attack, harm, or threat to survival. Our autonomic nervous system automatically produces the adrenaline that helps us react quickly to the emergency.

But many people with MVPS/D can be in the physiological state of fight or flight *even when there is no danger present*. This is because their nervous system is out of balance and, therefore, may overreact to simple events by responding in precisely the same way as it would in the face of real danger.

For example, if your house was on fire, it would be perfectly appropriate for the fight or flight response to be activated. However, with a person who has MVPS/D, it may take just the bursting of a balloon to set off the fight or flight response. This stimulus, the bursting of the balloon, although seemingly innocuous, can set off exactly the same kind of physiological changes in someone with MVPS/D as if their house was on fire.

What Can I Do to Control My Stress?

You cannot eliminate all the stressful events in your life, but you can learn to control how you react to them. The antidote to the fight or flight condition is the "relaxation response." Some relaxation techniques are briefly discussed below. A relaxation cassette by Mina

Soffer, of the Florida Institute for Cardiovascular Care can be helpful for some people (see Resources).

Breathing

One of the ways we respond to stress is by inadvertently holding our breath or with rapid, shallow, and irregular breathing. Unfortunately, most people breathe this way most of the time. Yet as newborns we all breathed from our abdomens. Abdominal breathing is a simple and powerful stress management technique.

To practice abdominal breathing, sit comfortably with your back straight. Place your right hand on your abdomen and place your left hand on your chest. This will help you to be aware of your abdominal muscles as you breathe. Concentrate on contracting your diaphragm and breathing from deep within your abdomen. As you inhale, push out your abdomen.

Practice this breathing, making sure your exhalation is twice as long as your inhalation. Always breathe through your nose to filter and warm the air and exhale gently through your mouth. You can test whether you are breathing properly by lying on the floor and placing a telephone book on your abdomen. If you can see the book rise up when you inhale and lower when you exhale, you are breathing correctly.

Progressive Muscle Relaxation

Muscles that tense up in response to anxiety often don't fully relax even after the stress is gone. When someone is in a state of chronic stress, these muscles remain constantly tight. There is a powerful and effective technique to relax the muscles by successive tensing and relaxing of the voluntary muscles in an orderly sequence until all the main muscle groups of the body are relaxed.

By using progressive muscle relaxation you can learn to recognize the difference between how your muscles feel when they are tensed or relaxed and you can learn how to release the tension before it manifests itself into a headache or backache.

In the following exercise, you may want to work with just one set of muscle groups for about five minutes, or you may want to do a full twenty-minute workout and work with all the muscle groups.

Tense It and Then Release It

- Hands: Tense your fists; relax. Extend your fingers; relax.

- Biceps and triceps: Tense the biceps; relax. Tense the triceps; relax.

- Shoulders, chest, and back: Take a deep breath; hold it. Your shoulders should be pulled back hard. Tighten your chest muscles at the same time; relax. Your shoulders should be pulled forward; relax.

- Neck: Roll your head slowly on your neck's axis three times. Do the same in the other direction.

- Mouth: Open your mouth as wide as possible; relax. Purse your lips in an exaggerated pout; relax.

- Tongue: Extend your tongue as far as possible; relax. Bring your tongue back into your throat as far as comfortably possible; relax.

- Eyes and forehead: Close your eyes and imagine something or someplace enjoyable.

- Midsection: Raise your midsection slightly by tensing your buttock muscles; relax.

- Stomach: Pull your stomach in as hard as possible; relax. Extend your stomach; relax.

- Calves and feet: Tense the muscles in the calves and feet; relax.

- Toes: Stretch your toes toward you; relax. Bend your toes in the opposite direction; relax.

Experiment with the different relaxation techniques. Some people find it difficult to meditate and prefer progressive muscle relaxation, while still others prefer abdominal breathing to relieve stress. Do whatever works best for you.

Meditation

Meditation has always been a part of most cultures and religions. It is simply a way of quieting your mind. When your mind is quiet, you feel peaceful and whatever stress you might be feeling, diminishes and ultimately disappears. You can meditate anywhere and at any time. It is best to find a quiet environment and begin by focusing on your breathing. Allow your body to relax each time you exhale.

To practice meditation, you begin by focusing your mind on one thing at a time. For example, you could light a candle and focus on the candle flame, trying not to think of anything but just looking at the flame and staying aware of your breathing. At first, you probably will find that your mind wanders. All sorts of thoughts may come to you. Acknowledge them and then let them go. Don't follow the thoughts. If you find yourself thinking about something in detail, remind yourself that you are not there to think, but to meditate and to focus on quieting your mind. If your mind wanders, pay attention to your breathing instead of to the thoughts on your mind.

You might find that focusing on a word, phrase, or sound instead of focusing on a candle works better to quiet your mind. You could repeat words to yourself, words such as, "joy," "love," "happiness," or phrases like "I am at peace." This is called a *mantra*. You can repeat your mantra over and over again.

This repetition is an effective way of focusing your mind and preventing distracting thoughts. Additional ways to meditate are by taking the time to "stop and smell the roses" and allowing your senses to enjoy nature by listening to ocean waves, enjoying the nearest park, or watching the sunset. Although simple, these methods have proven effective in the treatment of MVPS/D (Soffer, *A Patient's Guide*, 1999).

Visualization or Guided Imagery

Visualization is similar to meditation. It's the technique of using your imagination to focus on and create positive conscious and unconscious attitudes for relaxation and well-being. The power of imagination can create a very real physical response. We are all born with imagination. Our bodies can respond right away to mental images as if we were really where we are imagining ourselves to be.

Many athletes use visualization to improve their performances by creating mental pictures of their desired goals, as if those goals had already been achieved, or by visualizing and rehearsing their improved performance step-by-step.

When you practice visualizing vivid mental imagery, you can create pictures of your body repairing and healing itself. If you practice visualizing these images often enough and deeply enough, you will be sending powerful signals to your subconscious mind about getting well.

Your subconscious mind is very powerful, and harnessing those powers is the intent of practicing visualization exercises. Today, there are many books about visualization and many courses taught on how best to do it. One excellent book, by Pat Fanning, is called *Visualization for Change* (2001).

Spirituality

Some people use the words "spiritual" and "religious" interchangeably, but spirituality is really a much broader, more encompassing term. Religious ideas and concerns are only part of a much larger concept. So, although some people's spirituality is very much related to God or a higher power and might include organized worship in a church, synagogue, or mosque, for others, spirituality may have nothing to do with organized religion and going to church. For example, meditating, playing and listening to music, and focusing on nature can all be spiritual activities. The following activities might help you to begin or continue your journey into spirituality:

- Try meditating.

- Find an accessible church, synagogue, or mosque and see if it meets your spiritual needs. Places of worship provide strong spiritual and social support to people with a variety of physical, emotional, and spiritual needs.

- Volunteer to help those who need help. You could volunteer for a religious organization or for another type of nonprofit organization. Can you tutor reading? Can you help out with a breakfast program? Can you visit the sick people in hospitals who have no family or friends?

- Read books on spirituality and meditation, or find audiotapes on those subjects. If you have a computer and Internet access, look for sites that deal with spiritual concerns.

- Develop some spiritual disciplines. These might include prayer groups, Bible reading, Bible study, or group meditation.

- Find a support group or a network of people who have similar concerns or problems.

- Pray. Focus on your relationship with God, your family and friends, and your needs and concerns.

- Talk to your doctor about your physical and spiritual needs. You might be surprised about his or her openness to spiritual needs.

Laughter

Whether it's a tiny giggle or an all-out belly-busting whoop, laughter makes life a lot easier. By looking at the humorous side of life, you shift your focus away from the stress of a situation, clearing the way for stress relief. Laughter initiates the release of beta-endorphins, those same natural relaxants that are released during exercise. Endorphins make you feel good and protect your immune system by blocking cortisol, an immune system suppressor. If you tend to take yourself too seriously, recruit help. Call a friend who makes you laugh or rent a comedy at the video store.

Until more is known about mitral valve prolapse syndrome/dysautonomia and more research is done, it will continue to remain a controversial subject. In the meantime, people who know they have, or believe they have MVPS/D cannot sit back and wait for the controversy to be settled as to whether it is a full-blown syndrome, or not. They are looking for help.

This book was written to help those of you who are suffering from MVPS/D or who know someone who is suffering from MVPS/D. We hope it has enlightened you and helped you to cope with your symptoms. More importantly, we hope it has made you realize that you are not alone and that you are not "going crazy."

Turning MVPS/D into a Positive Strong Point

I always tell people that having MVPS/D is the best thing that ever happened to me. A lot of them look at me in disbelief, until they realize that I am telling the absolute truth.

I, myself, didn't always believe this to be the truth, until I started working on improving my MVPS/D symptoms. Working on conquering fears and phobias is not always easy, but when I began to conquer mine, I also began to see how most "normal" people take life for granted.

Life for me had been so difficult for so many years, that once I started recovering from panic disorder, I began to stop and smell the roses. In fact, I even started feeling sorry for people who cannot appreciate the little things in life.

People who get upset about traffic, delays at the airport, slow service at a restaurant, and so on, don't realize that they take for granted driving, flying, and being out in crowds. They don't understand how happy they should be that they are able to live the quality of life they want for themselves. They haven't figured out that traffic jams, delays at the airport, and slow restaurant service are, at most, nothing more than minor annoyances, meaningless in the grand scheme of things.

Having MVPS/D has changed my whole perspective on life. You can do the same things you did before you had it. You may not believe that at this very moment, but once you begin to get your nervous system back in balance, you will have the opportunity to look at life from a different perspective. I urge you to take advantage of this opportunity. I appreciate that life is wonderful, and that there is a lot of enjoyment to be had in it; there is a lot that I intend to accomplish.

You, too, can accomplish whatever it is you wish to accomplish. Get your nervous system back in balance and there will be nothing that can slow you down again.

—Cheryl L. Durante

Resources

Anxiety Disorders of America
11900 Parklawn Drive, Suite 100
Rockville, MD 20852-2624
301-231-9350
www.adaa.org

Bio Bright, Inc.
Light therapy for SAD
7315 Wisconsin Avenue, Suite 1300
Bethesda, MD 20814-3202
800-621-LITE

Center for Coping
www.coping.com
Robert H. Phillips, Ph.D.

Endometriosis Association
8585 N. 76th Place
Milwaukee, WI 53223
800-992-3636
www.endometriosisassn.org

Exercise and Fatigue
www.mylifeguardforhealth.com

Fear of Flying
www.anxieties.com

Florida Institute for Cardiovascular Care
Mitral Valve Prolapse Center
3700 Washington Street, Suite 300
Hollywood, FL 33021
Ariel D. Soffer, M.D., Director
954-967-6550 or 877-96-HEART
www.mitral.com
Audiotape: "Relax and Manage Your Stress," Mina Soffer, M.S., L.M.H.C

Freedom From Fear
308 Seaview Avenue
Staten Island, NY 10305
718-351-1717

Headache Help
www.headache-help.org

International Foundation of Gastric Disorders
Irritable bowel, GERD, and other G.I. disorders
www.aboutibs.com

Mental Health FAXU
301-443-5155
Listen to recorded instructions to receive, by fax, a listing of free articles.

Mental Health Net
www.mentalhealth.net

MVPS Information
www.mediscene.com
Al Davies, M.D.

The Mitral Valve Prolapse Center of Alabama
880 Montclair Road, Suite 370
Birmingham, AL 35213
Phillip C. Watkins, M.D., Director
205-592-5765
800-541-8602
www.mvprolapse.com

The Mitral Valve Prolapse Society
(A nonprofit, charitable organization)
P.O. Box 431
Itasca, IL 60143
630-250-9327
Fax 630-773-0478
Bonnie0107@aol.com
www.mitralvalveprolapse.com
Bimonthly newsletter (pen pal listing)

National Fibromyalgia Partnership
140 Zinn Way
Linden, VA 22642
866-725-4404
www.fmpartnership.org

National Institute of Mental Health (NIMH)
6001 Executive Boulevard
Room 8184, MSC 9663
Bethesda, MD 20892-9663
800-421-4211
www.nimh.nih.gov

National Society for Mitral Valve Prolapse and Dysautonomia
Baptist Hospitals Foundation
P.O. Box 830605
Birmingham, AL 35283-0605
205-592-5765

Northern Light Technology (Canada)
514-335-1763
Fax 514-335-7764

Panic Disorder
http://panicdisorder.about.com

The Scoliosis Association
P.O. Box 811705
Boca Raton, FL 33481
800-800-0669
www.scoliosis-assoc.org

The Springhill Memorial Hospital MVP Clinic
3719 Dauphin Street
P.O. Box 8246
Mobile, AL 36608
251-461-2438
800-923-2656

The Sun Box Company
19217 Orbit Drive
Gaithersburg, MD 20879
800-LITE-YOU

Tinnitus Association
www.tinnitus.com

Tinnitus Device
Aurex 3
201-767-6040
Fax 201-784-0620

The Tinnitus Relief System CD
800-551-4467

The TMJ Association, Ltd.
6418 W. Washington Boulevard
Wauwatosa, WI 53231
414-259-9334
www.tmj.org

University of Washington
Frederick A. Matsen, M.D.
Orthopaedics and Sports Medicine
www.orthop.washington.edu

Your Heart Health
www.heartcenteronline.com

Recommended Books

The Antidepressant Survival Program
Robert J. Hedaya, M.D.
Crown Books

The Anxiety Disease
David V. Sheehan, M.D.
Bantam Books

Confronting Mitral Valve Prolapse Syndrome
Lyn Frederickson, R.N., M.S.N.
Warner Books

On the Edge of Darkness: Conversations About Conquering Depression
Kathy Cronkite
Doubleday Company

The Good News About Depression
Mark S. Gold, M.D.
Villard Books

Headache HELP
Lawrence Robbins, M.D., and Susan S. Lang
Houghton Mifflin Company

Natural Therapies for Mitral Vlave Prolapse
Ronald L. Hoffman
M.D. Keats Publishing Company

Winter Blues: Seasonal Affective Disorders
Norman E. Rosenthal, M.D.
The Guilford Press

Support Groups

Austin, TX
> Mary Lou Dupuis
> 512-636-4781
> mid@austin.rr.com

> Margaret Hoffer
> 512-246-1032
> Hoffer@ev1.net

Birminham, AL
> Christi Wilson
> 205-621-2055
> clfoo73@cs.com

Centreville, VA
> Elly Brosius
> 703-968-9818
> EleanorBB@aol.com

Hendersonville, NC
Diane Stepkoski
828-692-6246
dstepkoski@a-o.com

Itasca, IL
MVPS Society
630-250-9327
Fax 630-773-0478
bonnie0107@aol.com

Pasadena, CA
Catherine Thomas
626-798-3466

Sheldon, IL
Hazel Harris
815-429-4003
h-harris45@hotmail.com

References

Abben, R. A. No date. Personal communication.

Bourne, E. J. 2001. *Beyond Anxiety and Phobia: A Step-by-Step Guide to Lifetime Recovery*. Oakland, CA: New Harbinger Publications.

The American College of Obstetricians and Gynecologists. 2000. Guidelines on diagnosis and treatment of PMS. *The American Journal of Gynecology*: 52-61.

Corder, R., J. A. Douthwaite, D. M. Lees, N. Q. Khan, A. C. Viseu dos Santos, E. G. Wood, et al. 2001. Endothelin-1 synthesis reduced by red wine. *Nature News Service* 414:863-864.

Cotton, E. 1992. Stress and headaches. *MVP Update*, Fall issue, p.1

Dajani, A. S., K. Taubert, W. Wilson, A. F. Bolger, A. Bayer, P. Ferrieri, et al. 1997. Prevention of bacterial endocarditis. *American Heart Association Scientific Statement* 96:359-362.

Davies, A. 1996. The syndrome. *And The Beat Goes On*. Itasca, IL. March/April issue, pp.1-2.

————. 1995. *A Guide for Patients: Mitral Valve Prolapse (MVP) Dysautonomia*. Houston, Texas: Baylor College of Medicine and the Methodist Hospital.

Davis, M., E. R. Eshelman, and M. McKay. 2000. *The Relaxation & Stress Reduction Workbook*. Fifth edition. Oakland, CA: New Harbinger Publications.

Devereux, R. B., C. J. Frary, R. Kramer-Fox, O. W. Isom, J. S. Borer, M. J. Roman, et al. 1994. Cost-effectiveness of infective endocarditis prophylaxis for mitral valve prolapse with or without a mitral regurgitant murmur. *American Journal of Cardiology* 74(10):1024-1029.

Eiken, T. 1991. Sleep disorders and the MVP patient. *Prolapse Potpourri*. Spring issue, p.1.

Fanning, Pat. 2001. *Visualization for Change.* Second edition. Oakland, CA: New Harbinger Publications.

Ford, R., and K. Ford. 1996. Migraine is associated with mitral valve prolapse: But that doesn't mean you have to suffer. *MVP Upbeat* 7:1-2.

Frederickson, L. 1992. *Confronting Mitral Valve Prolapse Syndrome.* Second Edition. New York: Warner Books.

———. 1992. When panic attacks. *Prolapse Potpourri.* Complimentary issue, p. 5.

Freed, L. A., D. Levy, R. A. Levine, M. G. Larson, J. C. Evans, D. L. Fuller, et al. 1999. Prevalence and clinical outcome of mitral valve prolapse. *The New England Journal of Medicine* 341(1): 1-7.

Gilliland, R. 1997. MVP and fibromyalgia. *And the Beat Goes On.* Itasca, Illinois. September/October issue, pp.1-2.

Greist, J., J. Jefferson, and I. Marks. 1986. *Anxiety and Its Treatment.* New York: Warner Books.

Hamilton, R. 1997. Subscriber's page. *And The Beat Goes On.* Itasca, IL. July/August issue, p. 3.

———. 1991. Panic disorder. The most frequently reported psychiatric syndrome associated with MVP. *Prolapse Potpourri.* Fall issue, pp. 1-2.

Hedaya, R. B. 2000. *The Antidepressant Survival Program.* New York: Crown Publishers.

Hoffman, R. L. 1997. *Natural Therapies for Mitral Valve Prolapse.* New Canaan, CT: Keats Publishing.

Luketic, R., and L. Watkins. 2000. 50 health-improving reasons to exercise. *MVP Upbeat.* Winter issue, p.4.

MVP Center of Birmingham, Alabama. 1993. What effect does salt, too much or not enough of, have on MVP? *MVP Update.* Spring issue, p.2.

———. 1990. Symptoms commonly associated with the presence of mitral valve prolapse. *Prolapse Potpourri.* Summer issue, p.1.

———. 1989. What is mitral valve prolapse? *Prolapse Potpourri.* Complimentary issue, p. 1.

———. 1987. Special dietary considerations for the MVP patient. *Patient brochure* from The Mitral Valve Prolapse Center of Alabama, p.3.

Mulumudi, M. S., and K. Bivekananthan. 2001. Mysteries of mitral valve prolapse: proper treatment requires consideration of all clues. *Postgraduate Medicine* 110:2.

National Institute of Mental Health. 1999. *Facts About Generalized Anxiety Disorder.* Bethesda, MD. Booklet No. OM 99-4153.

———. 1995. *Understanding Panic Disorder.* Bethesda, MD. Booklet No. NIH 95-3509.

Phillips, R. 1992. *Coping with Mitral Valve Prolapse.* Garden City Park, NY: Avery Publishing Group.

Preston, J., J. O'Neal, and M. Talaga. 1999. *Handbook of Clinical Psychopharmacology for Therapists.* Second edition. Oakland, CA: New Harbinger Publications.

Rippetoe, P. 1997. Medication phobia—allaying the fears. *MVP Upbeat.* Fall/Winter, pp. 4-5.

———. 1993. *The Psychology of Mitral Valve Prolapse and Panic Attacks.* Booklet from the Southeastern Conference on Mitral Valve Prolapse, Birmingham, AL. p. 97.

Roach, M. 1998. A quick fix for fatigue. *Health Magazine.* October issue, pp. 62-65.

Rosenthal, N. 1993. *Winter Blues: Seasonal Affective Disorder, What It Is and How to Overcome It.* New York: The Guilford Press.

Rowe, P. C., H. Calkins, and J. Kan. 2002. Suggestions for a high sodium diet. Department of Medicine, Johns Hopkins Hospital. www.medjhu.edu

Russell, R. O., Jr. 1993. The History of MVP Syndrome. Paper presented at the Southwestern Conference on Mitral Valve Prolapse on May 15, 1993, at the Jefferson Civic Center in Birmingham, Alabama.

Sacher, M. 2000. Heart-healthy diet. Heart Center Online. www.heartcenteronline.com

Sargent, M. 1994. *Depressive Illnesses: Treatments Bring New Hope.* National Institute of Mental Health. Bethesda, MD: Booklet No. NIH 94-3612.

Sawyer, N. 1991. Beta-blockers. *Prolapse Potpourri.* Spring issue, p. 2.

Singh, R. G., R. Cappucci, R. Kramer-Fox, M. J. Roman, P. Kligfield, J. S. Borer, et al. 2000. Severe mitral valve regurgitation due to mitral valve prolapse: Risk factors for development, progression, and need for mitral valve surgery. *American Journal of Cardiology* 85(2):193-198.

Soffer, A. 1999. A common goal. *MVP Upbeat.* Summer issue, p.1-2.

———. 1999. *Mitral valve prolapse: A patient's guide to a healthier, happier life.* Florida Institute for Cardiovascular Care. Patient Guide, pp.15-18.

Starlanyl, D., and M. Copeland. 2001. *Fibromyalgia & Chronic Myofascial Pain.* Second edition. Oakland, CA: New Harbinger Publications.

Starlanyl, D. 1999. *The Fibromyalgia Advocate.* Oakland, CA: New Harbinger Publications.

Sullivan, D. 2001. Exercise and fatigue. Consumer Health Interactive (CHI), partners with mylifeguardforhealth.com. Online Web site.

Utter, A. C., J. Kang, and R. J. Robertson. 2001. Perceived exertion. *Current Comment from the American College of Sports Medicine.* August issue, p. 1.

Watkins, P. 1998. Exercise and depression. *MVP Upbeat* 7:1.

——— 1997. Treatment of symptomatic mitral valve prolapse syndrome and dysautonomia. *Cardiology in Review* 5:4.

———. 1995. Better living with mitral valve prolapse. *MVP Upbeat* 7:7.

———. 1990. Holiday blues. *Prolapse Potpourri.* Winter issue, p. 2.

Watkins, P., and R. Russell. 1990. Mitral valve prolapse syndrome: Appropriate diagnosis is key to a happy patient. *Illustrated Medicine* 5:2.

———. 1990. Mitral valve prolapse syndrome: Appropriate diagnosis is key to a happy patient. *Illustrated Medicine* 5:9.

Weidenbach, K. 2000. Exposure therapy explored for treatment of driving phobias. *Stanford University News Report.* July 12, 2000 issue, p. 1.

Wolfson, A. R. 2001. *The Woman's Book of Sleep.* Oakland, CA: New Harbinger Publications.

James F. Durante is the president of The Mitral Valve Prolapse Society. He was diagnosed with MVPS in 1990. **Cheryl L. Durante**, a cofounder of the Mitral Valve Prolapse Society, was diagnosed with MVPS in 1988. They both live in Itasca, Illinois.

John Gerard Furiasse, MD, is a cardiologist and director of cardiac rehabilitation at Alexian Brothers Medical Center, Elk Grove, Illinois and is the president of Cardiovascular Associates also in Elk Grove, Illinois.

Some Other
New Harbinger Titles

Stop Worrying Abour Your Health, Item SWYH $14.95

The Vulvodynia Survival Guide, Item VSG $15.95

The Multifidus Back Pain Solution, Item MBPS $12.95

Move Your Body, Tone Your Mood, Item MBTM $17.95

The Chronic Illness Workbook, Item CNIW $16.95

Coping with Crohn's Disease, Item CPCD $15.95

The Woman's Book of Sleep, Item WBS $14.95

The Trigger Point Therapy Workbook, Item TPTW $19.95

Fibromyalgia and Chronic Myofascial Pain Syndrome, second edition, Item FMS2 $19.95

Kill the Craving, Item KC $18.95

Rosacea, Item ROSA $13.95

Thinking Pregnant, Item TKPG $13.95

Shy Bladder Syndrome, Item SBDS $13.95

Help for Hairpullers, Item HFHP $13.95

Coping with Chronic Fatigue Syndrome, Item CFS $13.95

The Stop Smoking Workbook, Item SMOK $17.95

Multiple Chemical Sensitivity, Item MCS $16.95

Breaking the Bonds of Irritable Bowel Syndrome, Item IBS $14.95

Parkinson's Disease and the Art of Moving, Item PARK $16.95

The Addiction Workbook, Item AWB $18.95

The Interstitial Cystitis Survival Guide, Item ICS $15.95

Illness and the Art of Creative Self-Expression, Item EXPR $13.95

Don't Leave it to Chance, Item GMBL $13.95

Call **toll free, 1-800-748-6273,** or log on to our online bookstore at **www.newharbinger.com** to order. Have your Visa or Mastercard number ready. Or send a check for the titles you want to New Harbinger Publications, Inc., 5674 Shattuck Ave., Oakland, CA 94609. Include $4.50 for the first book and 75¢ for each additional book, to cover shipping and handling. (California residents please include appropriate sales tax.) Allow two to five weeks for delivery.

Prices subject to change without notice.